Investigating Digital Crime

Investigating Digital Crime

Edited by

Robin Bryant
Canterbury Christ Church University, UK

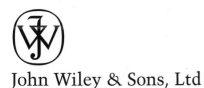

John Wiley & Sons, Ltd

Other Wiley Editorial Offices

John Wiley & Sons Inc., 111 River Street, Hoboken, NJ 07030, USA

Jossey-Bass, 989 Market Street, San Francisco, CA 94103-1741, USA

Wiley-VCH Verlag GmbH, Boschstr. 12, D-69469 Weinheim, Germany

John Wiley & Sons Australia Ltd, 33 Park Road, Milton, Queensland 4064, Australia

John Wiley & Sons (Asia) Pte Ltd, 2 Clementi Loop #02-01, Jin Xing Distripark, Singapore 129809

John Wiley & Sons Canada Ltd, 6045 Freemont Blvd, Mississauga, Ontario, L5R 4J3

Wiley also publishes its books in a variety of electronic formats. Some content that appears in print may
not be available in electronic books.

Library of Congress Cataloging-in-Publication Data

Investigating digital crime / edited by Robin Bryant.
   p. cm.
  Includes bibliographical references and index.
  ISBN 978-0-470-51600-3 (cloth) – ISBN 978-0-470-51601-0 (pbk.)
1. Computer crimes–Investigation. 2. Commercial crimes–Investigation.
I. Bryant, Robin, Dr.
HV8079.C65I59 2008
363.25'968–dc22

                                          2008012121

British Library Cataloguing in Publication Data

A catalogue record for this book is available from the British Library

ISBN 978-0-470-51600-3 (H/B)
ISBN 978-0-470-51601-0 (P/B)

Typeset in 10.5/13pt Times by Aptara Inc., New Delhi, India
Printed and bound in Great Britain by Antony Rowe Ltd., Chippenham, Wiltshire

Contents

Preface

Robin Bryant

Extensive media coverage, numerous government and industry reports and frequent police warnings have all contributed to a heightened awareness of new criminal opportunities following in the wake of the rapid growth of digital technologies. If we are not quite yet living in Castells' (1996) 'network society' we are, in many key respects, close to it. Superficially at least, it might appear that we have entered a new era with new forms of criminality. However, on closer examination, many of these supposedly novel forms of crime (such as phishing in order to perform an identity fraud) in fact share much in common with conventional and long standing crimes and criminal techniques. Thus the reader will encounter an ongoing debate throughout this book concerning just how 'new' are they, in reality, these 'new technology' crimes? This debate culminates in a chapter concerned with some of the developing criminological and motivational perspectives on digital crime.

In the chapters that follow, we have deliberately chosen to extend the discussion beyond the realms of what may be termed 'conventional cybercrime' (despite the apparent inherent contradiction of the phrase) to other forms of criminality that exploit digital technologies to a lesser or greater extent. Hence we examine telecommunications fraud, video game piracy and 'chip and PIN' credit and debit cards, in addition to considering well-recognised problems such as cybercrime and internet grooming. It is for this reason that we have adopted the phrase 'digital crime' within the title of the book.

This book examines the legislative and investigative response to digital crime both in chapters exclusively devoted to this subject, but also more generally throughout the remaining chapters. Given the international nature of much digital crime the discussion of legislation also extends to the European Commission's Convention on Cybercrime.

Digital crime will undoubtedly continue to present the law enforcement community with new investigative challenges, particularly of a technical nature, and we have attempted to delineate these challenges alongside a description of current law enforcement practice. The professional backgrounds of the contributors to this book, drawn from the academic community (particularly computer science), police training and criminal investigation, reflect this desire to engage with the issues surrounding investigation.

A rapid pace of change creates an ever-present danger for the authors of a printed work exploring the impact of new technologies; the book could well be out of date by the time it is published. It is inevitable that when you read this text, at least some of the crimes we examine will have faded from public consciousness, and drifted down the priority lists of digital crime investigators. We have tried to head off this danger by attempting to draw conclusions of a more lasting nature, based upon observations of current (and perhaps more transient) forms of criminal activity, but illuminated by theoretical perspectives.

Each chapter concludes with a set of questions for the reader, either as a review of the material covered or as questions to stimulate further research into the topics.

Acknowledgements

The authors would like to thank Detective Constable Paul McLea from the Police Service of Northern Ireland for his invaluable advice on the legal issues surrounding encryption legislation in the UK; Ed Day for providing feedback on earlier drafts of a number of chapters, Sofia Graca for translation, Karen Preece and Gill Lennon for proofreading Chapter 3; Emily Wilkins for her help in the final proof-reading and finally, Katy and Emily Stephens for their patience, support and understanding whilst several of the chapters were being produced by Paul Stephens.

Reference

Castells, M. (1996) *The Information Age: Economy, Society and Culture. The rise of the Network Society.* **1**: Oxford: Blackwell Publishers.

List of Contributors

Robin Bryant is Head of Department of Crime and Policing Studies at Canterbury Christ Church University. He has edited and contributed to several books on police training and published and presented widely on investigative theory.

Sarah Bryant specialises in redrafting and editing academic material of a technical nature for a wider readership. Her academic background is in science education and the development of learning materials for adults. She has contributed to the editing of all of the chapters, and also created and developed a number of diagrams and other aids to understanding in this book.

Joe Carthy is a Senior Lecturer and Director of the Centre for Cybercrime Investigation at University College, Dublin. Joe has published widely on cybercrime investigation and computer security and is the author/co-author of 70 scientific papers and a textbook on computer architecture.

Denis Edgar-Nevill is Head of Department of Computing at Canterbury Christ Church University. He led the development of the MSc Cybercrime Forensics which is jointly validated and delivered with the NPIA.

Paul Gillen is a Detective Inspector within the Garda Bureau of Fraud Investigation, Dublin. Paul is also currently the Project Manager of the EU Agis programme 'Cybercrime investigation – delivering an intermediate level accredited modular international training programme'.

Tahar Kechadi is a Senior Lecturer at the School of Computer Science & Informatics at University College, Dublin. His research interests span the areas of parallel processing, parallel architectures, security of parallel computing, multi-stage interconnection networks, heterogeneous distributed systems, scheduling, dynamic load balancing, artificial neural networks, optimisation techniques and Grid computing.

Ian Kennedy is a forensic computer analyst within the Digital Forensics Unit of Kent Police, south-east England. In addition to his operational police commitments, he is also a regular guest speaker at digital forensics lectures and the author of numerous articles published both in print and on the internet.

Angus Marshall is a Senior Lecturer in Forensic Science at the University of Teesside where he is responsible for the digital evidence portfolio. He is also a practicing expert witness for prosecution and defence. He is notorious for crashing deadlines and the mere mention of his name makes editors quail. His real passion is motoring, quickly, in classic sports and GT cars.

Dave O'Reilly is a consultant in the area of computer networks and IT security, application development and project management. He has designed and supervised implementation of business IT systems for clients around the world. Dave teaches occasional courses on computer network technology. On several occasions he has advised the Garda Siochana as an expert on computer networking.

Paul Stephens is Programme Director for the BSc (Hons) Forensic Computing programme at Canterbury Christ Church University. He has worked with, and taught, representatives of law enforcement agencies from across the European Union on digital crime related issues.

Tracey Stevens is Deputy Head of Hi-Tech Crime Training at the National Policing Improvement Agency. For the past five years she has specialised in the development and delivery of training both nationally and internationally for those involved in investigating digital crime. She has contributed to a number of Best Practice Guides issued to law enforcement agencies in this specialised area of work, including guidance for managers of high tech crime units and for those searching for and seizing digital evidence.

All views expressed represent those of the contributors and not necessarily those of their employers.

All trademarks, product names, company names or logos cited herein are the property of their respective owners.

1

The Challenge of Digital Crime

Robin Bryant

In this chapter we examine the challenges arising from the growth of digital crime, particularly the problems faced by investigators. The interaction between technological change and criminality is well recognised for crime in general, but certain aspects of digital crime mark a significant shift both in the ways in which crime is enacted, and the consequent investigative response. This chapter explores some of the more general technological and social factors that have accompanied and possibly contributed to these changes. The remaining chapters consider particular aspects in more detail.

1.1 Technology and crime

Throughout history, general technological developments have continually created new opportunities for criminal activity, which in turn have driven the development of new technologies. Both the pre-modern and modern eras provide clear examples of such interactions. For example, in the 12th century, the techniques employed for counterfeiting currency closely matched the technological development of reliable methods to produce genuine currency. Similarly, bank robbers in the early 20th

Investigating Digital Crime   Edited by Robin Bryant and Sarah Bryant
© 2008 John Wiley & Sons, Ltd

century soon began to use motor cars to speed their getaway, a scenario portrayed frequently in early Hollywood gangster movies such as *White Heat*. More recently, criminals employ advanced technology in their attempts to access internet-based banking systems in order to launder the proceeds of criminal enterprises.

The burgeoning development of a wide range of new technologies provides an ever expanding range of options for the creative mind. Some of the terminology relating to these technologies and their applications are shown in figure 1.1; no doubt digital crime investigators will already be familiar with the meanings of many of the terms shown.

Just as technology is utilised by many people for legitimate reasons, so it will be by those intent on committing crime. In this sense, little has changed; *plus ça change, plus c'est la même chose*. However, in the late modern age, crime that specifically exploits digital technologies (what we term in this book 'digital crime') has a number of possibly novel characteristics, and we explore these below.

1.1.1 Spatial and temporal differences

It perhaps now a cliché to observe that digital crime respects no international or legislative boundaries. However, it is undoubtedly true that much digital crime (particularly crime associated with the internet) is not anchored in time and space in quite the same sense as more conventional crime. Whereas the 1950s con artist inviting passers-by to 'Find the Lady' (pick out the Queen of Hearts from a row of three face-down playing cards) in London's Petticoat Lane would need to make direct personal contact to carry out the fraud, an eBay fraudster is not so constrained. Likewise, some crimes (such as installing a 'Trojan horse' virus) may be enacted in seconds, but the effect may not be felt until days, months or years later. Vatis (2005) goes so far as to claim that cybercrime in particular represents

> [...] the most fundamental challenge for law enforcement in the 21st century. By its very nature, the cyber environment is borderless, affords easy anonymity and methods of concealment and provides new tools to engage in criminal activity.

For digital crime, temporal differences are also significant, particularly in relation to the rapidity of interactions, such as receiving reward and gratification. The probable motivation for a person to illegally download the mp3 version of

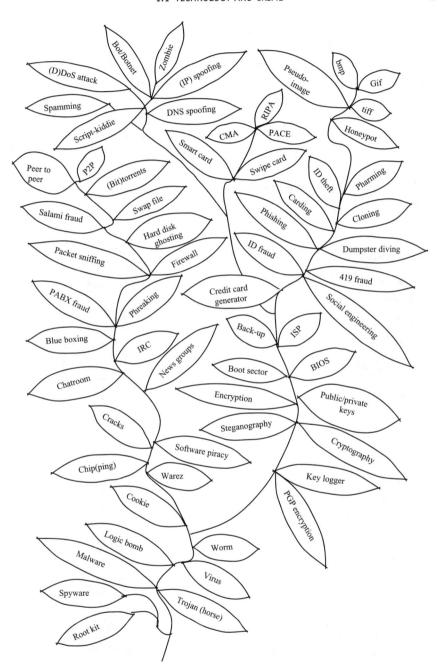

Figure 1.1 Digital terminologies (*Sarah Bryant*)

copyrighted music is not solely because it is relatively free of charge, but also because it is immediately available.

Access to information is no longer so constrained by time and space. It is far more difficult, largely as a result of the internet, for groups, organisations, authorities and official bodies to control access to certain forms of information, many of which may be considered to be sensitive or even dangerous. Once Pandora's digital Box is opened it is almost impossible to track down and remove any information released. On reflection, this should not be surprising, given the

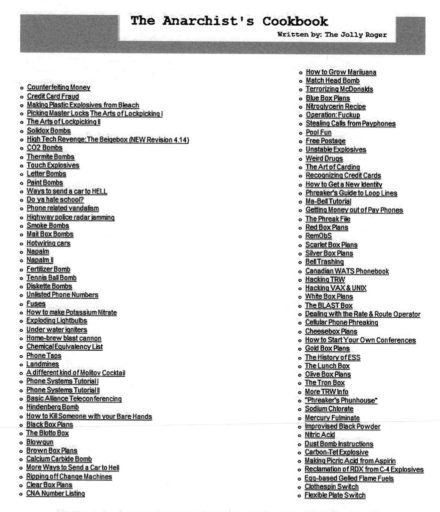

Figure 1.2   A typical hypertext version of the 'Anarchist's Cookbook'.

origins of the internet as a network designed to withstand attack. Contrast two documents produced in the 1970s: the so-called 'Green Book' produced by members of the Provisional IRA (to help train their recruits in the use of lethal weapons and quasi-military tactics) with the notorious 'Anarchist's Cookbook', a text still circulating on the internet which details, inter alia, the manufacture of improvised explosive devices.

Most of the 'military' content of the Green Book was strictly controlled and 'analogue' in nature (presumably mainly photocopied and distributed on paper), and has not apparently been released into the public domain. However, the Anarchist's Cookbook and similar documents (such as the Terrorist's Handbook) have been developed and expanded by a number of contributors working independently and anonymously (now as part of a wider project termed the 'Jolly Roger Cookbook') and are readily available to anyone through the internet. In 1999 David Copeland (not believed to be a member of any terrorist organisation) used information contained in the Terrorist's Handbook to construct nail bombs which he used to attack people in a gay bar in Soho in London, and then passers-by in Brick Lane and Brixton, both multi-cultural areas of London (BBC, 2000).

1.1.2 Economies of scale

Second, digital crime often exploits the ability of ICT to disseminate information widely, repeatedly and cheaply. As a result, what we might term the 'sucker quotient' for digital crime can be much lower than for conventional crime; for digital crime the investment of time and effort may be low, but the activity may still nonetheless provide high returns for the criminal. Our 1950s con artist is counting on quite a few people from those hundreds passing by to be gullible enough to take part in the con; the sucker quotient has to be relatively high for the con to yield sufficient results. On the other hand, a phisher can send tens of thousands of fake emails relatively easily, and even if only one victim responds, the resulting user account details may be used subsequently to commit identity theft and fraud, potentially very lucrative crimes. In a somewhat similar way, the pattern of rewards from other digital crimes follows the related principle of many victims and small losses. As Wall (2004, p. 20) suggests

> Where once a robber might have had to put together a team of individuals [...] in order to steal £1 million from a bank, new technologies are powerful enough (in principle at least) to enable one individual to rob one million people of £1 each.

1.1.3 Anonymity

Third, digital crime, particularly if it is conducted over the internet, provides a much greater scope for anonymity, through either secrecy or by presenting a false identity (DiMarco, 2003). A paedophile may brazenly assume a faked identity (perhaps as another young person) in an attempt to groom a potential victim in an online chatroom. In comparison, grooming in the pre-internet era necessitated the paedophile gaining the trust of the child and family by an often slow and (for the paedophile) risky face-to-face process.

1.1.4 Virtual worlds

Fourth, the virtual nature of some digital crime (Brenner, 2001) is an important explanatory and defining factor. In a very loose sense this refers to the sense of unreality or even 'de-individualisation' (akin to Zimbardo's concept of 'deindividuation') with an attendant loss of sense of self-accountably and self-awareness pervading a person's actions in the digital world, particularly online. This sense of unreality may in turn lead to disinhibition (Suler, 2004). For example, many people make no attempt to conceal the fact that they have committed the theft of intellectual property online (using peer-to-peer programs (P2P) to download copyrighted music), but they would otherwise consider themselves to be entirely law-abiding citizens (Yar, 2007).

1.1.5 Legislative lag

Fifth, digital crime (particularly cybercrime) is perceived to suffer from an increased propensity to 'legislative lag'; a longer period of time seems to elapse between innovations in criminal enterprise and the response of the state and law enforcement agencies. This is probably an illusion; digital crime develops and changes very rapidly, but it may take years for legislation to be enacted, by which time the crime may well have mutated or developed to assume a different form. In consequence, it may seem that many digital crimes are in effect beyond the reach of law, and indeed this may be the case; at least some digital crimes cannot be addressed under contemporaneous legislation. This is a complex area, discussed more fully in later chapters, but it is interesting to note at this stage that the UK government does not share the view that specific e-related legislation is always necessary, or that there is necessarily a problem of legislative lag:

> The Government is committed to ensuring that actions should be legal or illegal according to their merits, rather than the medium used, i.e. what is illegal offline should be illegal online and vice versa. As such, all legislation criminalises offences regardless of the means used to commit the offence.
>
> Where there is a need to revise legislation to take account of new criminal techniques we seek to do so. We liaise regularly with the prosecution and law enforcement authorities to ensure the criminal law remains fit for purpose, but are not aware of significant legislative gaps that hinder the agencies (Home Office, 2006).

1.1.6 Horizontal and vertical hierarchies

Using an analogy with the four kinds of mapping employed in mathematical set theory, we can conceptualise the main forms of human communication as falling into one or more categories, as illustrated in Table 1.1.

Table 1.1 Mapping forms of communication

Form of communication (mapping)	Hierarchy	Example
One-to-one	Predominantly horizontal (across)	Person to person, e.g. by speaking or writing a letter
One-to-many	Predominantly vertical (downwards)	One person addressing a group, e.g. making a speech to a group of people
Many-to-one	Predominantly vertical (upwards)	A group of people addressing one person, e.g. a written petition to a politician
Many-to-many	Predominantly horizontal (across)	Groups of people communicating with others, e.g. a 'Facebook' entry on the internet

It is in the many-to-many forms of communication that we have probably witnessed the most significant change as a result of digital forms of data storage and communication. As Dupont (2004) notes, the advent of the internet in particular has led to the 'decline of vertical hierarchical social structures and the concomitant rise of horizontal networks'. That is, in the past, the flow of some forms of information tended to be 'top down' and hence under the control of those occupying a higher position in a hierarchy. This applied as much to knowledge concerning criminal matters as it did to more socially acceptable forms of information.

Horizontal structures, particularly single horizontal planes from a much larger vertical hierarchical pyramid, also tend to be less efficient in terms of opportunities for communication. Communication is often limited to a relatively small group of people within the horizontal plane, leaving a silent and unempowered majority; a scenario that may be familiar to employees within large organisations. There are other examples; incarceration in prison is sometimes an opportunity for criminals to share information concerning criminal techniques, such as improved ways to commit a burglary (Gill, 2007). However, given the nature of the information concerned it was by necessity limited to a small circle, (and be largely verbal in nature) and would as a consequence spread only slowly.

If we accept that the internet has led to an increase in horizontal communication, that is amongst peers with little or no control exercised by authorities, then this will also be reflected in new opportunities to share information and techniques amongst those interested, or intent upon, criminal activities. There is some patchy evidence that this may be happening. For example, it is alleged that the notorious US-based 'Shadowcrew' online community (located around the now closed website

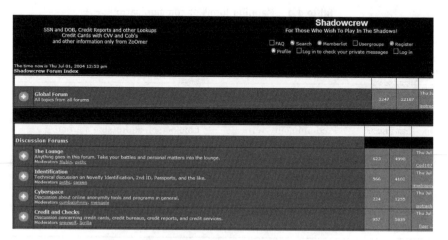

Figure 1.3   Excerpt from the 'Shadowcrew' website in 2004

www.shadowcrew.com) shared and traded information concerning stolen credit card numbers and ATM skimmers, and it is claimed that these activities resulted in the loss of $4 million, (United States of America v. Mantovani and others, 2004). At its height it is alleged that the Shadowcrew community consisted of over 4000 members (United States of America v. Mantovani and others, 2004).

1.1.7 Investigative challenges

Finally, by its very nature digital crime can give rise to a number of specific detection and investigative challenges. For example, the use of steganography to hide child pornographic images can pose the kind of technical and legislative problems inconceivable just two decades or so ago. Steganography is the process of hiding one object within another. It predates the digital era; Allied PoWs concealed messages in letters written to loved ones, using barely visible dots (amongst other means). However, interest in steganographic techniques has received an added impetus for two main reasons; its use to hide electronic information (such as a child pornographic image within an innocent-looking holiday snap) and the wide availability of software to assist the process. Note that steganography is not simply cryptography in a different guise: in the use of cryptography for example, it is obvious that a change has been made to the original information, with steganography it is not.

There are well-documented cases of the use of steganography by criminals, such as the sharing or selling of child pornography. For example, in 2002 an international police investigation ('Operation Twins', led by the UK's NHTCU and involving Europol, the Canadian RCMP and police forces from Norway and Germany) uncovered an extensive paedophile ring whose members frequently employed steganography to hide child pornographic images. Less well substantiated is the claim that the technique is also used by terrorists. Gabrielle Weimann, a senior fellow at the United States Institute of Peace and Professor of Communication at Haifa University claimed in March 2004 that:

> Hamas activists in the Middle East, for example, use chat rooms to plan operations and operatives exchange e-mail to coordinate actions across Gaza, the West Bank, Lebanon, and Israel. Instructions in the form of maps, photographs, directions, and technical details of how to use explosives are often disguised by means of steganography. (Weimann, 2004)

Undoubtedly, the use of steganography presents a serious challenge to digital investigators (McBride *et al.*, 2005), and for a number of reasons. For example,

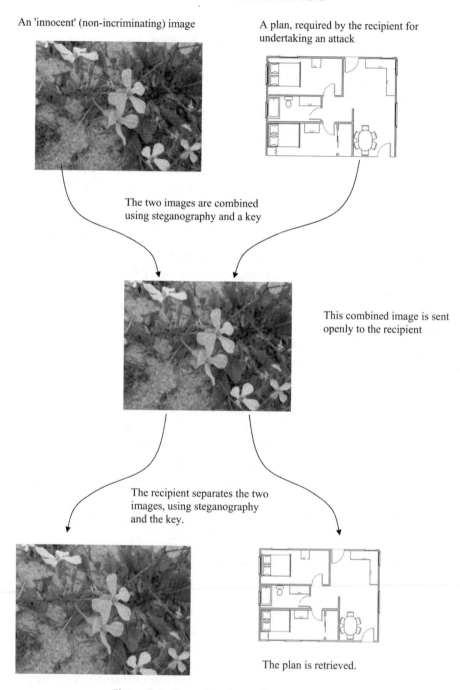

An 'innocent' (non-incriminating) image

A plan, required by the recipient for undertaking an attack

The two images are combined using steganography and a key

This combined image is sent openly to the recipient

The recipient separates the two images, using steganography and the key.

The plan is retrieved.

Figure 1.4   Concealing images by steganography

by deliberate intent, steganographic versions of illegal images are impossible to identify simply by sight, and sophisticated techniques are necessary for both identifying the existence of a file changed through steganography and in recovering the original in a manner that would withstand legal scrutiny (steganalysis). Often the hidden file is password protected and forms of cryptography can also be used as part of the steganographic process, adding another level of difficulty for the investigator.

1.2 Analogue and digital

In popular culture we are often said to live in a 'digital world', presumably a reference to those information and communication technologies (the internet, the mobile phone), consumer and entertainment products (DVD, satellite TV) which exploit the advantages of storing and transmitting data represented in a *digital* form. The term digital used in this context probably arose from the word digit, referring to the fingers, particularly when used in counting (*digitus* is Latin for a finger or toe). Increasingly, digital has come to mean the representation of information (in its most fundamental form) as a number of states, usually two states, but sometimes three or more. Two-state systems are sometimes termed as binary, referring to states such as '1' and '0' or 'on' and 'off'. This is not a new idea; the reliability of such systems is exploited in Morse code which uses a two-state representation of dots and dashes, (although intervals of four different lengths are used to help decode messages). According to the *Oxford English Dictionary* (2007) the more modern sense of the word 'digital' first came into use in 1984.

Digital technology is often contrasted with precursor analogue (or analog) technologies. Analogue technology represents information in a form that is analogous to the quantity or quality itself. Perhaps the classic example of this is the difference between analogue watches (using the movement of hands to represent the time), and digital watches which use only numbers. We can draw an analogy between position and time for the hands of an analogue watch; the hands move through space at a rate proportional to the lapse of time. In this way, an analogue watch attempts to replicate the phenomenon of time itself by a direct copying; the smooth movement of the hands representing time as a continuous variable. Digital watches use a more abstract representation instead, identifying points in time such as 10:23, with the passage of time itself not represented visually. The time will then appear to suddenly move on, to 10:24, 10:25 and so on; time is represented as if it is a discrete variable.

Music and other sounds may also be stored by analogue or digital means. A comparison of earlier analogue methods (the acetate or vinyl record) and later digital approaches (the CD) provides a further illustration of some key differences between analogue and digital representations. Consider two copies of the Beatles' Sgt Pepper album, one a vinyl LP, the other a CD. On the vinyl disc the spiral groove is visible (just), with its variable peaks, troughs and gradients; complex shapes that are analogous to the sounds produced when the disc is played. On the other hand, the sound on a CD is represented as digital data; physically this consists of only a series of simple 'pits' and 'lands'; a two-state representation (invisible to the unaided human eye).

Sound recordings

The line represents the groove on a vinyl record, as seen from above, for a mono record.

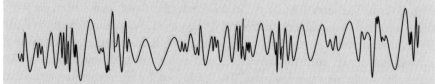

Figure 1.5   A representation of a groove on a vinyl record

The wider the sideways displacement of the groove, the louder and deeper the sound. Higher pitched sounds are carried by tightly packed oscillations. For a stereo recording, the width of the groove itself varies too, allowing the stylus to move up and down as well as from side to side.

The diagram below shows the simple way in which information is represented digitally as 'pits' and 'lands', as seen from above.

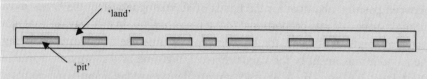

Figure 1.6   A representation of part of a digital track on a CD

The dark areas are the pits (depressions) in the plastic surface. All the pits are the same depth; only the distance between them varies. The lands are the regions in between the pits. A laser moves along the track as the CD is read. The distance between successive pit-land transitions is the significant information in the signal.

Which format is likely to be illegally shared on the internet? The answer is obvious: the digital version, largely because the numerical representation of the pattern of pits and lands is far easier to reproduce than the precise and complex patterns engraved into the vinyl. The digital version also readily lends itself to conversion to other formats such as mp3, and to sharing through peer-to-peer networks. Crucially, because of the way that information is represented in a digital signal, there is no loss of quality when copying or sharing: the ten thousandth copy sounds exactly the same as the original.

The robustness of digital data also has significant advantages for data transmission. As the signal is composed of just two or more states, each relatively easily distinguishable from the other, it will remain clear and readable, almost regardless of the amount of distortion inadvertently introduced. As an example consider the developments in satellite TV broadcasting in the last decade or so. In the past, the satellite signal was essentially analogue in nature, and frequently subject to some distortion due to incorrectly aligned dishes, problems at the transmission end or weather conditions. Therefore, for the viewer, the picture might have been near perfect, or fuzzy with 'sparklies', or so fuzzy that there was almost no picture at all; the distortion in the signal created a proportionally distorted sound and picture. However, digital satellite signals (now the norm, at least for European and North American distributors) can still be 'read' accurately even if the signal is distorted, and the picture remains near-perfect. This is a slight simplification, as signal compression may produce a 'blocky' picture as the signal becomes more distorted, and of course complete picture loss is inevitable if the signal is so severely distorted that the states become indistinguishable. For the same underlying reason, messages in Morse code may remain clear, even if the signal has been transmitted over thousands of miles, as the code contains only six elements that are relatively easy to distinguish.

The storage of information in digital form also facilitates the integration of devices and systems. Whereas in the past a personal phone could not play music, and a tape deck was not an answering machine, now the distinction between the functionality of digital devices (particularly those designed for the consumer market) is increasingly blurred, and deliberately so. A mobile phone might well also function as a GPS device and a DVD player might also be able to show digital photographs. Some refrigerators even have IP addresses on the internet.

The differences between analogue and digital means of storage and repro-duction may appear to be largely technical in nature but these differences are important when attempting to understand the nature of digital crime. For exam-ple, the increased availability and distribution of hardcore adult pornography have been greatly facilitated by the use of digital media. In the 1970s and 1980s, VHS tapes of hardcore pornography originating from countries where its production and trade were legal could only be distributed to other countries to a limited ex-tent, partly due to technical difficulties in producing multiple copies. A VHS tape copied 'serially' (that is, making copies of copies) is virtually unwatchable after at most three or four copies, due to compounded errors in reproduction. However, digital formats can be serially copied without any loss of information, so produc-tion of such material is now far easier, and can be carried out successfully on a smaller scale.

Not only do these changes in forms of distribution affect crime but they also influence legislative and regulatory responses; indeed the censors' apparently more liberal views may be to some extent a pragmatic response to the widespread availability of hardcore pornography through digital media, resulting in desensi-tisation. In the case of adult pornography, the British Board of Film Classification (BBFC) now allows most forms of adult hardcore pornography (images of aroused genitalia and ejaculation) to be sold from licensed sex shops in the UK. However, the BBFC's decision (as a result of a High Court decision) must also be viewed against the wider context of changes of attitude to censorship.

Finally, digital data occupies far less physical space than its analogue equiv-alents. For example, a novel of 125 000 words would probably cover about 500 paper pages, but could be stored digitally in a volume much smaller than a pinhead, occupying about 1.25 Mb in digital terms. Similarly, 128 000 such novels could be stored on a single 160 Gb PC hard drive. The digital storage 'space' required can be reduced still further through the use of encoding and compression tech-niques. For example, an average CD audio track occupies between 50 to 60 Mb, but can be compressed to about four Mb when encoded in mp3 format, and for most listeners there will be no noticeable loss of quality.

1.3 The growth of digital technologies

The telephone was the first mass-market two-way communication device. The first public telephone exchange (serving only eight subscribers) was opened in 1879 (BT, 2007), but it was not until the mid 1970s that more than 50 per cent of the households in England and Wales had their own landline telephone. And from the

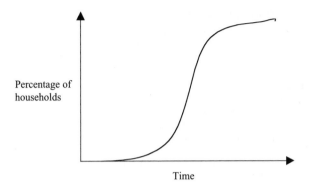

Figure 1.7   Market penetration of new products

1922 inception of regular radio broadcasting by the BBC, it took almost 30 years for radio to become a regular presence in almost every home. Most new consumer devices follow a characteristic 'S' shape of take-up, as illustrated in Figure 1.7.

In the early years of a new device (e.g. the 'wireless' radio) take-up is relatively slow (the lag phase) but then gains pace before slowing again; at this stage market penetration may approach (or even exceed) 100 per cent for some items.

This 'S' shaped pattern of consumer behaviour has also been observed for many new (digital) technology devices but with a noticeable difference: the 'S' shape is often much more foreshortened with a more rapid acceleration towards market adoption. For example, it was estimated that in 2006, 57 per cent of households in Great Britain had an internet connection with 73 per cent of these being broadband, compared with just nine per cent in 1998 (National Statistics Online, 2006).

Not only has there been an exponential growth in the numbers of digital devices in circulation and the number of digital services utilised; the processing power of digital devices has increased dramatically. Moore's Law, originally formulated in the mid 1960s observed that the number of transistors in an integrated circuit doubled every two years, but that the real cost remained constant year after year, (Intel, 2007). In popular use Moore's Law has now assumed a more general meaning, and is often used (perhaps erroneously) to make the case that processing power doubles every 18 months to two years. Certainly, technological advances have given rise to cheap and widely-available computing power in a wide variety of forms. The consequences of such rapid technological change (and its implications for crime) are difficult to predict, but are likely nonetheless to be real and manifest.

For example, the cost of many digital devices has decreased significantly in the last decade or so, as illustrated by the Table 1.2. The power and functionality of these devices has also increased.

Table 1.2   The changing costs of digital devices

Device	Cost in 1997	Cost in 2007
Mid-range desktop PC	£1200	£400[1]
Basic DVD player	£275	£14.98[2]
'Entry level' mp3 player	£180[3]	£14.99[4]

[1] Ebuyer, http://www.ebuyer.com/UK/store/5/cat/Home-PCs
[2] Tesco, Bush 2051ND DVD Player, http://direct.tesco.com/q/R.100–1141.aspx
[3] The first portable mp3 players appeared in 1998.
[4] Play.com, Inovix IMP-15 256MB MP3 / WMA Player, http://www.play.com/Product.aspx?r=
ELEC&title=1063434&source=9710

At the present time, the cost of digital devices is still falling and their functionality and power is increasing; it may seem paradoxical that a convergence of
technologies is coinciding with increased specialisation. For example, even an
'entry level' PC will play a music collection, and many mobile phones will also
take photographs, however it becomes more of a challenge for the average person
to make simple repairs to his or her own car. Digital services are also increasingly
being 'bundled' together (Ofcom, 2007) leading to a greater convergence and
take-up of digital television, broadband and VoIP.

At the same time, digital devices are tending to become smaller whilst remaining consistent with practical use, referred to in the past as miniaturisation. For
example, mobile phones were the size of a house brick until the 1990s and a DVD
player is likely to be slimmer and much lighter than its equivalent predecessor,
the VCR (partly because it has far fewer moving parts). As we see in section 1.6
below, these reductions in size have implications for digital crime.

The growth in digital technologies and their widespread and rapid adoption
(including information communication technologies) have obviously provided
new opportunities to commit crime; these crimes and the investigative response
are the subjects of most of this book. However, microprocessors and storage
memory in many devices (other than the usual locations such as PCs and PDAs)
also provide new opportunities for investigators; additional forms of evidence,
and more sophisticated investigative methods and means for law enforcement.
For example, many new cars (particularly the higher specification models) come
equipped with GPS navigation devices which store data relating to locations
and times (and some of this information will not be apparent to the average
user). This information may be used as intelligence in an investigation or be
used as evidence in court. It may seem ironic that although a driver using a GPS
system may feel more independent, the device can also be used by others to track
movements retrospectively; this could be seen as a loss of independence as well

as a possible invasion of privacy. Of less obvious interest to the investigator (and less well known to the public) is the fact that some modern washing machines are equipped with ROM that may contain residual information concerning time of use; this could be important, for example, in an investigation into an alleged rape. In essence, whenever a digital device contains memory it is of potential interest to an investigator.

1.4 Key features of digital crime

In popular discourse, in crime investigation and within the academic community, a number of terms are used relating to the advent of new (or 'retooled') forms of criminality associated with the growth of digital technologies (see Section 1.3 above). These terms include 'new technology crime', 'cybercrime' and 'high

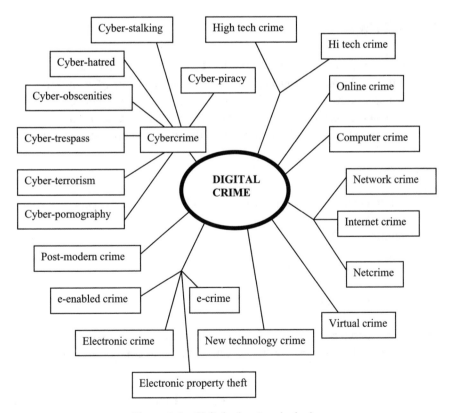

Figure 1.8 Digital crime terminologies

(or 'hi') tech crime'. In addition, the prefixes 'e' and 'cyber' also tend to be attached to existing labels to indicate new and 'digitised' versions of existing crime phenomena.

Wall (2004) argues the need for accurate terminology when describing these new forms of crime. It is debatable therefore, whether we really need yet another term, such as 'digital crime' to describe some of these phenomena. However, digital crime is more than cybercrime (Wall, 2005, 2007 (Chapter 2)), e-crime (cited by Morris, 2004), netcrime, new technology crime, online crime, high tech crime. The term 'digital crime' embraces most of these, but also includes other forms of crime, such as music and video piracy, which have grown and developed largely as a consequence of the growth of digital technologies and the opportunities for criminal enterprise that we examined in the preceding section. As Kshetri (2005, p. 555) notes: 'Crimes target sources of value, and for this reason, digitization of value is tightly linked with digitization of crime'.

Cybercrime

More recently, the term 'cybercrime' has taken on a more defined meaning, and this is reflected in a growing literature on the subject. Cybercrime is increasingly being defined as that crime which occurs in a networked environment (such as the internet), and which is peculiar to these environments.

The term cybercrime usually embraces the following criminal activities:

- computer hacking and cracking;

- developing and/or spreading malicious code (e.g. virus, Trojans);

- spamming;

- network intrusion;

- software piracy; and

- network-based or network-enabled crimes such as phishing, identity theft, IPR crimes (e.g. illegal filesharing), distribution of child pornography.

However, we acknowledge that such a wide meaning for digital crime results in a somewhat tautological or 'catch all' definition. In this sense we are closer

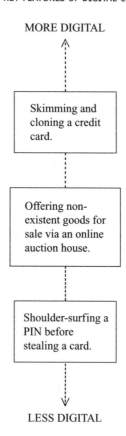

Figure 1.9 The digital spectrum

to Grabosky (2007, p. 2) who uses the term 'electronic crime' to describe 'a wide range of crimes committed with the aid of digital technology', but, like ourselves, also acknowledges that this is a 'label of convenience'. Wall (2005) proposes the application of an 'elimination test' to a crime – that is, if we ignore the digital features of a crime, has a crime still been committed (or has the crime been 'eliminated')? Wall goes on to suggest that crimes can be placed along a spectrum depending on the extent of digital involvement; some crimes may involve only incidental use of a computer, whilst other crimes, such as phishing, could not be committed without computers and computer technology. It is the crimes at this latter end of the spectrum that we might conceptualise as digital in nature, if not form. Figure 1.9 shows some examples of crimes and their positions along this spectrum.

Consider a street thief who first observes an unwary user input their PIN at an ATM, and then steals the card and later withdraws cash; this is not a crime that appears to be particularly digital, and it is therefore placed at the less digital end of the spectrum. On the other hand, skimming the magnetic stripe of a credit card, cloning the card, and then using it to make transactions is clearly a crime unique to the digital era, and would appear to be placed at the more digital end of the spectrum.

However, many crimes are more likely to have a digital aspect rather than to uniquely exploit digital technologies. An example would be a fraud enacted via an online auction house such as eBay (see Figure 1.8 above); this type of fraud belongs to the long and dishonourable tradition of separating the gullible from their money, and there would appear to be little that is 'post – or even late – modern' about it. However, the fraudster may well have undertaken planning for the fraud involving the internet; setting up temporary and difficult to trace email accounts and surfing the internet for images, descriptions and prices. Furthermore, he or she may well have falsified his or her own 'satisfaction rating' to inspire confidence in sellers, and then bid on his or her own fake auction, using a 'shill' account to up the price. These are all activities which exploit the advantages of digital technologies, but nonetheless arise from a conventional and classic form of crime.

1.5 Growth and development of digital crime

As we noted in the introduction to this chapter, changes in technology (particularly forms of information communication) almost always provide new opportunities for crime. However, although there may be new opportunities and ample evidence of individuals exploiting these opportunities for illegal gain, it will not necessarily lead to an overall increase in criminal activity. An important question therefore, is how much of this new crime is simply a displacement or reconfiguration of previous criminal activity? Or has there been a genuine increase in overall levels? This is a complex issue; as an illustration, consider the impact of digital technologies on copyrighted music and video and intellectual property rights crime.

In the 1960s it was just about possible to copy music using consumer-level equipment, but the process was technically demanding and far from reliable; reel-to-reel tape machines were expensive and the process involved using a microphone to record from the radio or a vinyl record onto a tape. The whole approach was thoroughly analogue in nature, and normally produced only a single taped copy of listenable quality. Though (to our knowledge) no academic research has been undertaken on this particular issue, home taping of copyrighted music by amateur enthusiasts seems not to have been considered a problem in the 1960s, and certainly not by the companies that may potentially have been affected.

Home taping of film images (largely 8 mm film stock) was (if anything) at an even earlier stage of development than taping music in the 1960s. There were no consumer VHS or Betamax recorders available to copy from TV, and most piracy at this time consisted of copying film (often pornography) for private distribution, and was limited to those with access to specialist equipment.

In the 1970s and 80s, with the advent of relatively inexpensive audio cassette players with a record button, home taping of copyrighted popular music became widespread, and came to be perceived as problematic, particularly by the record producing industries. For example, in the early 1980s the British Phonographic Industry (BPI) organisation launched their 'Home Taping is Killing Music' campaign. At about the same time, organised counterfeiting of music for criminal profit became widespread; commercially-produced copyrighted music (on tape or vinyl) was copied (in parallel and in series) onto tapes for selling on.

The first Betamax video player for the consumer market was introduced in the mid 1970s, but it could not make recordings (and cost over $2000). By the mid 1980s VHS had won the video format 'war' and video players and recorders became widely available. Inevitably these were used to make taped copies of commercially produced videos. One UK company even marketed a 'double-decker' VHS machine; tapes could be copied without the need for a second VHS deck. Despite its clear potential for making pirate copies, the House of Lords judgement (CBS Songs Ltd and Others v Amstrad Consumer Electronics Plc and Another, [1987] 2 WLR 1191) held that the company could not be held responsible for the misuse of the machine. Copy protection such as Macrovision was introduced, but so too were forms of circumvention (the 'signal cleaners' advertised in satellite, video and TV magazines).

Music CDs were introduced to the market in the early 1980s but it was not until CD recorders became widely available (initially as 'stand alone', then normally as part of a PC) that CD copying began in earnest. Before the internet became a widespread means of digital communication, this copying was usually 'physical', from one CD to another. Copies of commercial CDs were made by the owner of the CD as so-called 'back ups', or for passing or selling to another person. In most cases, the distribution of these copies was limited to a relatively small circle of friends, family and acquaintances. There were relatively few instances of organised physical piracy of CDs using specialised equipment to make numerous pirated CDs, but this began to increase in the late 1980s.

As in earlier decades, the digital piracy of visual media in the 1980s lagged behind music piracy. This was largely because video had not yet been digitalised to the same extent as music, and remained in analogue VHS format until the late 1990s. DVDs for the popular market became available in the late 1990s. Initially, DVDs were difficult to copy because of copy protection (usually employing the Content Scrambling System or CSS) and the huge volumes of data involved. For example, the 1999 commercial DVD of the Disney film 'A Bug's Life' was over 4 Gb in size (not including 'extras') but blank recordable DVDs for the public market were limited at the time to 3.95 Gb.

In the late 1990s 'personal digital piracy' emerged as a phenomenon, as distinct from earlier forms of organised physical piracy of cassette tapes and CDs, (Enders Analysis, 2003). Initially this was through usenet internet groups but latterly through Napster, now BitTorrent and P2P (peer-to-peer) successors, and involved the sharing of the mp3 versions of copyrighted music, and more latterly film and software. No physical piracy was required. This digital (or cyber) piracy became possible for a number of reasons:

- The increased speed of the internet through the rapid take-up of broadband, allowing much faster bit rates.

- A reduction in file size, using compression techniques with no major loss in auditory or visual quality. For example, the mpeg4 ('divx' or 'avi') version of the film 'Shaun of the Dead' is about one-tenth of the size of the original DVD; approximately 750 Mb compared to 7.63 Gb.

- A further reduction in file size, using software designed to 'strip out' extras such as alternative soundtracks and subtitling.

- The circumvention of copy protection, using programs such as DeCSS which became widely and freely available through the internet.

Both personal and physical digital piracy ('illegal filesharing' and 'commercial music piracy' or 'counterfeiting' respectively) are now considered to be serious problems by the companies and organisations involved. For example, the BPI claims that 'Illegal peer-to-peer filesharing has already had an enormous effect on British music sales; with an estimated £1.1bn in revenue lost in the last three years as a direct result' (BPI, 2007). However, as Wall (2007) and others note, the nature of online crime makes it difficult to accurately quantify statistics of this kind, and some industry-based organisations may have a particular interest in emphasising the seriousness of the problem.

1.6 A new criminology?

Many digital crimes can be understood and 'explained' in conventional criminological terms. For example, the miniaturisation of digital devices makes them more likely to be a target of crime, and their attractiveness to criminals can be understood, at least in part, through Clarke's familiar crime-reduction 'CRAVED' model (Clarke, 1999), as Table 1.3 illustrates.

However, what proportion of digital crime is actually new (in the sense of new forms of criminality) and how much is simply a modern manifestation of old (in some cases, ancient) and existing forms of crime? This issue has stimulated a lively academic debate, and as we alluded to earlier, is sometimes referred to as the '*plus ça change*' question, (from the French phrase '*plus ça change, plus c'est la même chose*' which may be translated as 'the more things change, the more they stay the same'.) For example, Hollinger (writing in 1997 on published research from 1976) noted that many of the early examples of 'computer abuse' were

Table 1.3 The CRAVED model and mobile phones

	Mobile phones pre 1990s (e.g. car phone)	Mobile phones 2007
Concealable	Typically up to 30 cm in length and hence not easily concealable	Easily concealable due to small size
Removable	Often fixed in some way inside a car	Rarely fixed, easily removable
Available	Rare	In many countries approaching or even over 100% market penetration
Valuable	Very expensive	A wide range of value
Enjoyable	Largely limited to business or other professional uses	Wide degree of functionality, added capability including mp3 playing, etc.
Disposable	Limited market for stolen mobiles	Vibrant market for second-hand mobiles, unofficial 'unchipping' services on offer

instead 'simply older forms of deviance and crime 'retooled' for the computer age' (Hollinger, 1997). Others argue that we are witnessing distinctly different and new forms of criminal behaviour, some of which can be attributed to the new ways in which we communicate and interact with one another. If there are distinctly new forms of criminal behaviour do we need matching new criminological theories? For example, David Wall outlines six commonly understood features of traditional criminal activity but concludes that 'In contrast, cybercrimes would appear to exhibit nearly the opposite characteristics' (Wall, 2005, p. 87).

Questions

Robin Bryant & Sarah Bryant

1. What activities illustrate the relationship between crime and technology in pre-modern eras?

2. What is 'deindividualisation' and how might this explain some online criminal behaviour?

3. 'Internet and other new digital crimes pose a challenge to those traditional criminological theories that emphasise the importance of place and time'. In what ways do we have to adjust our ways of thinking about crime and policing with the advent of information and communication technologies?

4. 'We should seek to distinguish between "true" cyber crime (i.e. dishonest or malicious acts which would not exist outside of an online environment, or at least not in the same kind of form or with anything like the same impact), and crime which is simply "e-enabled" (i.e. a criminal act known to the world before the advent of the worldwide web, but which is now increasingly perpetrated over the Internet).' (Burden & Palmer, 2003, p. 222).

5. How far is this distinction still valid?

References

BBC (2000) Nailbomber set out to 'terrorise'. BBC News [Online]. Available at: http://news.bbc.co.uk/1/hi/uk/782876.stm (Accessed: Oct 9 2007).

BPI (2007) Online music and the UK record industry. [Online]. Available at: http://www.bpi.co.uk/index.asp?Page=news/apu/news_content_file_825.shtml (Accessed: Oct 9 2007).

Brenner, S. (2001) Is there such a thing as virtual crime?. *Californian Criminal Law Review* **4**(1).

BT (2007) The historical development of BT. [Online]. Available at: http://www.btplc.com/Thegroup/BTsHistory/History.htm (Accessed: Oct 9 2007).

Burden, K., Palmer, C. (2003) Internet crime – cybercrime – a new breed of criminal? *Computer Law and Security Report 222* **19**(2):222–227.

Clarke, R.V. (1999), Hot Products: Understanding, Anticipating and Reducing Demand for Stolen Goods. (Police Research Series Paper 112) [Online]. Available at: http://www.homeoffice.gov.uk/rds/prgpdfs/fprs112.pdf (Accessed: Oct 9 2007).

DiMarco, H. (2003) The electronic cloak: secret sexual deviancy in cybersociety. In: Jewkes, Y. (ed.) *Dot.cons: Crime, Deviance and Identity on the Internet.* Cullompton: Willan Publishing.

Dupont, B. (2004) Security in the Age of Networks. *Policing & Society* **14**(1):76–91.

Enders Analysis (2003) Piracy Will it kill the music industry? [Online]. Available at: http://www.endersanalysis.com/enders/documents/Piracy%20ES%20(Ref%202003–12).pdf (Accessed: Oct 9 2007).

Gill, M. (2007) *Modus operandi of a thief conducted amongst 13 convicted British burglars.* Perpetuity Research and Consultancy International Ltd on behalf of Halifax General Insurance Ltd.

Grabosky, P. (2007) *Electronic Crime.* New Jersey: Pearson Education Inc.

Hollinger, R. (1997) Introduction. In: Hollinger, R. (ed.) *Crime, Deviance and the Computer.* The International Library of Criminology, Criminal Justice and Penology. Aldershot: Dartmouth.

Home Office (2006) Memorandum by the Government (Home Office and the Department of Trade and Industry). House of Lords Select Committee on Science and Technology, 29 November 2006 [Online]. Available at: http://www.parliament.the-stationery-office.com/pa/ld200607/ldselect/ldsctech/999/6112902.htm. (Accessed: Oct 9 2007).

Intel Corporation (2007) Moore's Law. [Online]. Available at: http://www.intel.com/technology/mooreslaw/ (Accessed: Oct 9 2007).

Kshetri, N. (2005) Pattern of global cyber war and crime: A conceptual framework. *Journal of International Management* **11**:541–562.

McBride, B., Peterson, G. and Gustafson, S. (2005) A new blind method for detecting novel steganography. *Digital Investigation* **2**(1):50–70.

Morris, S. (2004) The future of netcrime now: Part 1 – threats and challenges. (Home Office Online Report 62/04). [Online]. Available at: http://www.homeoffice.gov.uk/rds/pdfs04/rdsolr6204.pdf (Accessed: Oct 9 2007).

National Statistics Online (2006) Internet Access. [Online]. Available at http://www.statistics.gov.uk/CCI/nugget.asp?ID=8&Pos=1&ColRank=2&Rank=704 (Accessed: Oct 9 2007).

Ofcom (2007) Communications Market Report (23 August 2007) [Online]. Available at: http://www.ofcom.org.uk/research/cm/cmr07/cm07_print/cm07_1.pdf (Accessed: Oct 9 2007).

Suler, J. (2004) The Online Disinhibition Effect. [Online]. Available at: http://www.rider.edu/~suler/psycyber/disinhibit.html (Accessed: Oct 9 2007).

United States of America v. Mantovani and others (2004) [Online]. Available at: http://www.usdoj.gov/usao/nj/press/files/pdffiles/firewallindct1028.pdf#search=%22firewallindct1028.pdf%22 (Accessed: Oct 9 2007).

Vatis, M. (2005) statement to the Senate Judiciary Committee, Criminal Justice Oversight Subcommittee and House Judiciary Committee, Crime Subcommittee Washington, D.C. February 29, 2000, [Online]. Available at: http://www.usdoj.gov/criminal/cybercrime/vatis.htm (Accessed: 9 Oct 2007).

Wall, D. (2004) What are Cybercrimes? *Criminal Justice Matters* **58** Winter 2004/05: 20–21.

Wall, D. (2005) The internet as a conduit for criminals. In: Pattavina, A. (ed.) *Information Technology and the Criminal Justice System.* London: Sage Publications, pp. 77–98.

Wall, D. (2007) *Cybercrime.* Cambridge: Polity Press

Weimann, G. (2004) How modern terrorism uses the internet. [Online]. Available at: http://www.usip.org/pubs/specialreports/sr116.pdf (Accessed: Oct 9 2007)

Yar, M. (2007) Teenage kirks or virtual villainy? Internet piracy, moral entrepreneurship, and the social construction of a crime problem. In: Jewkes, Y. (ed.) *Crime Online.* Cullompton: Willan Publishing.

2

The Legislative Context for Digital Crime

Tracey Stevens

Throughout this book various areas of legislation are discussed in relation to specific aspects of digital crime and its investigation. In this chapter we examine computer misuse legislation and its development within the UK, with reference to new and amended Acts of Parliament, case law and other changes required under EU regulations. The following chapter should not be considered as an authoritative legal text, but rather as a guide to recent legislative changes enacted in response to new digital technology; how and why have particular pieces of new legislation come into being, and to what extent are the challenges presented by the criminal use of new technologies met?

Legislation often develops at a slower pace than technology (the legislative lag discussed in Chapter 1) and this can on occasion cause difficulties or be perceived as causing difficulties to those responsible for investigating offences involving digital technologies. However, it is also important to note that, even though the majority of current UK legislation was drafted prior to the digital age, most of it is still of relevance to the investigation and prosecution of digital crime.

Investigating Digital Crime   Edited by Robin Bryant and Sarah Bryant
© 2008 John Wiley & Sons, Ltd

2.1 International initiatives to combat digital crime

The international nature of digital crime and the consequent importance of harmonising national legal provisions have been widely recognised (Grabosky and Smith, 2001) and a number of initiatives have been made with an intention of increasing the potential for international cooperation. The Council of Europe's Convention on Cybercrime, considered to be a key point of reference, is one of the most comprehensive documents on cybercrime currently available. The Council aims to:

- harmonise the domestic criminal substantive law elements for offences (and connected provisions) relating to cybercrime;

- provide the powers for domestic criminal procedural law that are necessary for the investigation and prosecution of such offences (as well as other offences committed by means of a computer system or evidence in relation to which is in electronic form);

- help establish a fast and effective regime of international cooperation. (Convention on Cybercrime CETS No:185)

The offences defined by the Convention are illegal access, illegal interception, data interference, system interference, misuse of devices, computer-related forgery, computer-related fraud, offences related to child pornography and offences related to copyright and neighbouring rights. The Convention entered into force in 2004 and henceforth became a legally binding text. The full text of the Convention and its explanatory report are available on the Council of Europe's website (Council of Europe, 2001). By mid 2007, 21 countries had ratified the convention and 22 remained as signatories, the latter group including the UK.

In April 2002 a 'Proposal for a Council Framework Decision on attacks against information systems' was put forward by the European Commission. Its key aim was to encourage Member States to approximate rules on criminal law, and therefore to facilitate co-operation between judicial services (and other competent authorities) of separate member states.

The Convention on Cybercrime and the Framework Decision are closely connected and their definitions deliberately overlap. Table 2.1 provides a summary and comparison of the Articles of the Convention on Cybercrime and the Framework Decision with respect to standardising offences.

The Convention goes further than the Framework Decision as it deals with more than the creation of offences. In addition, the Articles of the Convention

Table 2.1   The Convention on Cybercrime and the Framework Decision

Convention on Cybercrime	Framework Decision on attacks against information systems
Illegal access (Article 2): Each party shall adopt such legislative and other measures as may be necessary to establish as criminal offences under its domestic law, when committed intentionally, the access to the whole or any part of a computer system without right. A party may require that the offence be committed by infringing security measures, with the intent of obtaining computer data or other dishonest intent, or in relation to a computer system that is connected to another computer system. *Illegal interception (Article 3):* Each party shall adopt such legislative and other measures as may be necessary to establish as criminal offences under its domestic law, when committed intentionally, the interception without right, made by technical means, of non-public transmissions of computer data to, from or within a computer system carrying such computer data. A party may require that the offence be committed with dishonest intent, or in relation to a computer system that is connected to another computer system.	*Illegal access to information systems (Article 2):* 1. Each member state shall take the necessary measures to ensure that the intentional access without right to the whole or any part of an information system is punishable as a criminal offence, at least for cases which are not minor. 2. Each member state may decide that the conduct referred to in paragraph 1 is incriminated only where the offence is committed by infringing a security measure.
Data interference (Article 4): 1. Each party shall adopt such legislative and other measures as may be necessary to establish as criminal offences under its domestic law, when committed intentionally, the damaging, deletion, deterioration, alteration or suppression of computer data without right. 2. A party may reserve the right to require that the conduct described in paragraph 1 result in serious harm.	*Illegal data interference (Article 4):* Each member state shall take the necessary measures to ensure that the intentional deletion, damaging, deterioration, alteration, suppression or rendering inaccessible of computer data on an information system is punishable as a criminal offence when committed without right, at least for cases which are not minor.

(Continued)

Table 2.1   (*Continued*)

Convention on Cybercrime	Framework Decision on attacks against information systems
System interference (Article 5): Each party shall adopt such legislative and other measures as may be necessary to establish as criminal offences under its domestic law, when committed intentionally, the serious hindering without right of the functioning of a computer system by inputting, transmitting, damaging, deleting, deteriorating, altering or suppressing computer data.	***Illegal system interference (Article 3):*** Each member state shall take the necessary measures to ensure that the intentional serious hindering or interruption of the functioning of an information system by inputting, transmitting, damaging, deleting, deteriorating, altering, suppressing or rendering inaccessible computer data is punishable as a criminal offence when committed without right, at least for cases which are not minor.
Attempt and aiding or abetting (Article 11): 1. Each party shall adopt such legislative and other measures as may be necessary to establish as criminal offences under its domestic law, when committed intentionally, aiding or abetting the commission of any of the offences established in accordance with Articles 2–10 of the present Convention with intent that such offence be committed. 2. Each party shall adopt such legislative and other measures as may be necessary to establish as criminal offences under its domestic law, when committed intentionally, an attempt to commit any of the offences established in accordance with articles 3 through 5, 7, 8, 9(1)(a) and 9(1)(c) of this Convention. 3. Each party may reserve the right not to apply in whole or in part, paragraph 2 of this article.	***Instigation, aiding and abetting and attempt (Article 5):*** 1. Each member state shall ensure that the instigation of, aiding and abetting and attempt to commit an offence, referred to in Articles 2, 3 and 4 is punishable as a criminal offence. 2. Each member state shall ensure that the attempt to commit the offence referred to in Articles 2, 3 and 4 is punishable as a criminal offence. 3. Each member state may decide not to enforce paragraph 2 for the offences referred to in Article 2.

also emphasise mutual assistance and international co-operation. A summary of the relevant Articles from the Convention is provided below:

Article 29 – Expedited preservation of stored computer data

A Party may request another Party to order or otherwise obtain the expeditious preservation of data stored by means of a computer system, which is located within the territory of that other Party and in respect of which the requesting Party intends to submit a request for mutual assistance for the search or similar access, seizure or similar securing, or disclosure of the data [the Article then details how a request is made and when it can be refused, etc.]

Article 30 – Expedited disclosure of preserved traffic data

Where in the course of the execution of a request made under Article 29 to preserve traffic data concerning specific communication, the requested Party discovers that a service provider in another State was involved in the transmission of the communication, the requested Party shall expeditiously disclose to the requesting Party a sufficient amount of traffic data in order to identify that service provider and the path through which the communication was transmitted [the Article continues with an outline of the circumstances where traffic data may be withheld.]

Article 31 – Mutual assistance regarding accessing of stored computer data

1. A Party may request another Party to search or similarly access, seize or similarly secure, and disclose data stored by means of a computer system located within the territory of the requested Party, including data that has been preserved pursuant to Article 29.

2. The requested Party shall respond to the request through application of international instruments, arrangements and laws referred to in Article 23, and in accordance with other relevant provisions of this Chapter.

Article 32 – Trans-border access to stored computer data with consent or where publicly available

A Party may, without obtaining the authorisation of another Party;

(a) access publicly available (open source) stored computer data, re-gardless of where the data is located geographically; or

(b) access or receive, through a computer system in its territory, stored computer data located in another Party, if the Party obtains the lawful and voluntary consent of the person who has the lawful authority to disclose the data to the Party through that computer system

Article 33 – Mutual legal assistance regarding the real-time collection of traffic data

1. The Parties shall provide mutual assistance to each other with respect to the real-time collection of traffic data associated with specified communications in its territory transmitted by means of a computer system. Subject to paragraph 2, assistance shall be governed by the conditions and procedures provided for under domestic law.

2. Each Party shall provide such assistance at least with respect to criminal offences for which real-time collection of traffic data would be available in a similar domestic case.

Article 34 – Mutual assistance regarding the interception of content data

The Parties shall provide mutual assistance to each other with respect to the real time collection or recording of content data of specified communications transmitted by means of a computer system to the extent permitted by their applicable treaties and domestic laws.

Article 35 – 24/7 Network

Each Party shall designate a point of contact available on a 24 hour, 7 day per week basis in order to ensure the provision of immediate assistance for the purpose of investigation or proceedings concerning criminal offences related to computer systems and data, or for the collection of evidence in electronic form of a criminal offence. Such assistance shall include facilitating, or, if permitted by its domestic law and practice, directly carrying out:

(a) provision of technical advice

(b) preservation of data pursuant to Articles 29 and 30; and

(c) collection of evidence, giving of legal information, and locating suspects.

The UK has not yet ratified the Convention on Cybercrime, but as a signatory has expressed its intention to become a Party to it. However, the UK is not bound by the signature and only becomes bound by the Convention at the point of ratification, at which stage the provisions of the Convention must be respected and implemented in full. Many of the articles of the Convention and the Framework Decision are already contained within the UK legal framework; indeed the precise wording of the articles of the Convention has been taken into account when changing UK legislation, helping promote compliance. A few further minor amendments to UK legislation are required in order to ensure full compliance, and it is likely that this will have been achieved by the time the Police and Justice Act 2006 comes into force; the UK will then be in a position to ratify.

2.2 Legal initiatives in the UK to combat digital crime

Several areas of legislation relating to digital crime have been amended or are in the process of being amended. Table 2.2 identifies the main Acts and sections of current legislation (within England and Wales) which are of specific relevance to digital crime. (There are some differences (not dealt with here) in respect of Scottish and Northern Irish legislation.) Note that many digital crimes are also covered under more general legislation concerned with theft and fraud. There are also a number of Statutory Instruments and EU Directives relevant to digital crime (not covered in this chapter).

Table 2.2 Legislation with specific relevance to the investigation of digital crime

---

Communications Act 2003
- s 125   Dishonestly obtaining electronic communication services
- s 126   Possession or supply of apparatus etc. for contravening S125
- s 127   Improper use of public electronic communication network

Computer Misuse Act 1990
- s 1   Unauthorised access to computer material
- s 2   Unauthorised access with intent to commit or facilitate the commission of a further offence
- s 3   Unauthorised modification of computer material

Copyright Designs and Patents Act 1988
- s 16   The acts restricted by copyright of a work, including copying
- s 17   Specifies the types of copy made, mentioning electronic storage
- s 107   Criminal liability for making or dealing with articles that infringe copyright
- s 110   Corporate liability for making copying equipment
- s 198   Criminal liability for making, dealing with or using illicit recordings

---

(Continued)

Table 2.2 *(Continued)*

Criminal Justice (Terrorism & Conspiracy) Act 1998
   s 5   Conspiracy to commit offences outside the UK

Criminal Justice Act 1988
   s 160   Possess an indecent photograph or pseudo photograph of child

Criminal Justice Act 2001
   s 50   Power to seize and sift

Data Protection Act 1998
   s 55   Unlawful obtaining of personal data

Forgery and Counterfeiting Act 1981
   s 10(3)   Inducing machines to accept a document as genuine

Malicious Communications Act 1988
   s 1   Offence of sending letters including 'electronic communication' to cause
             distress or anxiety

Mobile Telephones (Re-programming) Act 2002
   s 1   Changing the unique identifying characteristic of a mobile phone (the IMEI
             number)
   s 2 (1)   Owning the necessary equipment with the intent to use it for re-programming
             mobile phones
   s 2 (2)   Supplying the equipment
   s 2 (3)   Offering to supply the equipment

Obscene Publications Act 1959 and 1964
   s 2   Publish obscene article for gain
   s 2(1)   Storage and transmission of obscene material

Police and Criminal Evidence Act 1984
   s 18   Powers to search persons after arrest
   s 19   Powers of seizure, including hard copy print outs of information stored on
             computers
   s 20   Extension of powers of seizure to computerised information
   s 32   Searches of premises in which a person has been arrested

Protection from Harassment Act 1997
   s 2   Conduct amounting to harassment.

Protection of Children Act 1978
   s 1   Taking, making, distributing etc indecent photographs or pseudo photographs
             of a child

Public Order Act 1986
   s 21   Publishing or distributing material which is threatening or abusive or insulting
             if:
              • it is intended thereby to stir up racial hatred; or
              • having regard to all the circumstances, racial hatred is likely to be stirred
                thereby.

Racial and Religious Hatred Act 2006
s 29B   Using threatening words or behaviour, or displaying any written material
            which is threatening, if it is intended to stir up religious hatred.

Regulation of Investigatory Powers Act 2000
Pt 1, Ch I   Interception of communication
Pt 1, Ch II   Acquisition of communications data
Part III   Investigation of electronic data protected by encryption, powers to require
              disclosure (at the time of writing, not yet in force, but expected to take
              effect during October 2007)

Sexual Offences Act 2003
s 10   Causing or inciting a child to engage in sexual activity
s 11   Engaging in sexual activity in the presence of a child
s 12   Causing a child to watch a sexual act
s 14   Arranging or facilitating commission of a child sex offence
s 15   Meeting a child following sexual grooming, etc.

Terrorism Act 2000
s 1   Defines terrorism and includes acts designed to 'seriously disrupt an
            electronic system'

Copyright, etc. and Trade Marks (Offences and Enforcement) Act 2002
s 1   Criminal liability; illicit recordings, infringing articles and unauthorised
            decoders
s 2   Search warrants; illicit recordings and infringing articles and unauthorised
            decoders
s 3   Forfeiture of infringing copies and articles specifically for making copies
s 4   Forfeiture of illicit recordings and articles specifically for making copies
s 5   Forfeiture of unauthorised decoders

2.2.1 Computer Misuse Act 1990

The principal computer crime offences in the UK today are described within
the Computer Misuse Act 1990 (the CMA). The CMA was enacted following
recommendations by a Royal Commission, set up in response to difficulties arising
during prosecutions where the facts of a case (such as R. v. Gold and Schifreen
((1988) 2 WLR 984) could not be interpreted within the precise terms of the
existing legislation. Gold and Schifreen were hackers who had gained access to
the Duke of Edinburgh's computer files on the British Telecom Prestel Network.
At their original trial they were convicted of making a false instrument, an offence
under s 1 of the Forgery and Counterfeiting Act 1981. However on appeal, the
court held that the electronic impulses that formed the password could not be
considered to be an instrument within the definition of the Act. The House of
Lords overturned the convictions, agreeing with Lord Lane in the Court of Appeal

that there had been a 'Procrustean attempt to force the facts of the present case into the language of an Act not designed to fit them' (Wyatt citing Lane, (Hansard, 2005)).

The Criminal Damage Act 1971 is of limited use in cases involving modification or unauthorised access to computers, as in law it is held that it is not possible to criminally damage something that is not tangible. Under the Criminal Damage Act 1971, modifying the contents of a computer (or a computer storage medium) was not regarded as damage, unless the modification impaired its physical condition.

In 1991 however, a computer hacker was convicted under s 1 of the Criminal Damage Act 1971 in the case R. v. Whiteley ([1991] 93 Cr App R 25 (CA)). Whiteley had gained access to a computer network and altered data contained on disks in the system, causing the computer in question to be shut down for periods of time. It was held that:

> any alteration to the physical status might amount to damage within s 1 even though it was not tangible or perceptible to the human eye. The alterations of the magnetic particles on the disks and the impairment of their usefulness to the owner were sufficient.

The CMA is still a comparatively new Act compared with the majority of UK legislation, but it was drafted prior to many important technological breakthroughs. New devices and techniques (now familiar forms in the digital landscape) have inevitably presented new investigative and legal challenges; the CMA is in the process of being amended to ensure that it remains fit for purpose.

Procedure for amending the CMA

Part 5 of the Police and Justice Bill (introduced in the House of Lords in January 2006) relates to computer misuse, and contains proposed amendments to the existing CMA. In November 2006 the Bill received Royal Assent, becoming the Police and Justice Act 2006. However, the sections containing the amendments to the CMA are not yet in force.

The delay has been caused by the introduction of the Serious Crime Bill to the House of Lords in January 2007. The Serious Crime Bill contains amendments to part 5 of the Police and Justice Act 2006, and therefore the amendments to the CMA (proposed in the Police and Justice Act 2006) cannot come into force until the Serious Crime Bill has been enacted. The Serious Crime Bill has passed through the House of Lords but it is unlikely to have passed through Parliament and come into force until 2008.

Sections 1 and 2 of the CMA

Section 1 of the CMA relates to unauthorised access to computer material, commonly referred to as 'hacking'. Section 1(1) states (with future amendments in bold) that:

> A person is guilty of an offence if:
>
> (a) he causes a computer to perform any function with intent to secure access to any program or data held in any computer, **or to enable any such access to be secured**;
>
> (b) the access he intends to secure, **or to enable to be secured**, is unauthorised; and
>
> (c) he knows at the time when he causes the computer to perform the function that this is the case.
>
> S.1(2) The intent a person has to have to commit an offence under this section need not be directed at:
>
> > (a) any particular program or data:
> >
> > (b) a program or data of any particular kind; or
> >
> > (c) a program or data held in any particular computer.

Therefore, it is an offence to cause a computer to perform any function with intent to gain unauthorised access to a program or data held in a computer. To prove an offence, it has to be proved the computer access secured was unauthorised, and that the suspect knew the access was unauthorised.

It is important to appreciate the difference between gaining unauthorised access, and accessing a computer for an unauthorised purpose. These activities are different offences; the case of DPP v. Bignall ([1998] Cr. App. R. 1) clearly demonstrates the distinction. The defendants were charged with gaining unauthorised access to a computer, an offence contrary to s 1 of the CMA. The computer in question was the Police National Computer (PNC), and the charge was in fact wholly inappropriate for the circumstances; the defendants were police service employees, and were therefore fully authorised to access the system. However, the information gained from the computer system was subsequently used in an unauthorised way; the defendants could have been prosecuted under the Data Protection Act 1984 (now replaced by the Data Protection Act 1998).

The penalty for unauthorised access under s 1 of the CMA is imprisonment for up to 6 months or a fine, or both. It is a summary offence, therefore proceedings must commence within 6 months from the date the prosecutor feels there is sufficient evidence to prove the offence (Morgans v. DPP [1999] 1 W. L. R. 968). Section 35 of the Police and Justice Act 2006 (not in force at the time of writing) will make such unauthorised access an indictable as well as a summary offence, and increase the penalty for summary conviction.

Section 2 of the Computer Misuse Act 1990 covers unauthorised access to computers or computer systems (as for s 1), but with an additional factor; an intent to commit or facilitate further offences. There are no proposed amendments to this section, but it is included here for clarity. Section 2(1) states that:

> A person is guilty of an offence under this section if he commits an offence under s 1 above ('the unauthorised access offence') with intent:
>
> (a) to commit an offence to which this section applies; or
>
> (b) to facilitate the commission of such an offence (whether by himself or by some other person);
>
> and the offence he intends to commit or facilitate is referred to below in this section as the further offence.

A 'further offence' is an offence for which:

- the sentence is fixed by law; or

- a person of 21 years of age or over (not previously convicted) may be sentenced to imprisonment for a term of five years, or (in England and Wales) might be so sentenced but for the restrictions imposed by s 33 of the (1980 c. 43.) Magistrates' Courts Act 1980.

Under s 2, the activities in relation to a computer (or computer system) comprising an offence are the same as for s 1, but the s 2 offence is committed with the intention of committing a further offence, or facilitating the commission of a further offence. It is immaterial (for the purposes of this section) whether the further offence is to be committed on the same occasion as the unauthorised access offence, or on a future occasion. Even if the facts of the case are such that the commission of the further offence is impossible, a person may be still be guilty of an offence under this section if they had the intent to commit a further offence.

The penalty for a summary conviction under s 2 is up to six months imprisonment, a fine or both. For conviction on indictment, the penalty is up to five years imprisonment, a fine or both. If it is not possible to prove the intent to commit the indictable offence, the s 1 offence is still committed.

Section 3 of the Computer Misuse Act 1990

At present, s 3 of the CMA concerns unauthorised modification of computer material; a modification takes place if any program or data held on the computer is altered or erased, or if any new programs or data are added. (The offence is not about unauthorised access to a computer, so there is no necessity for any unauthorised access to have been obtained during the commission of the offence.) In some cases involving the disruption of computer systems, the existing s 3 of the CMA has been successfully used. However, the requirement for modification under s 3 of the CMA has caused problems; in some cases it has not been possible to prove that any modification has taken place.

The new s 3 will place more emphasis on impairing the operation of a computer. The entire s 3 of the original CMA is to be replaced under s 36 of the Police & Justice Act 2006. There are two main changes; a computer no longer has to be modified for an offence to be committed, and there will no longer be a requirement to prove intent; the acts can be committed recklessly.

Recently, there has been much discussion (and disagreement) between academics and lawyers as to whether or not Denial of Service (DoS) attacks fall within the existing s 3 of the CMA; have the data or programs on a computer been modified in any way during such an attack? Although prosecutions have been taken through the courts, defendants have usually been acquitted as a result of the 'Trojan defence' as opposed to the actual legality of charging someone under the existing s 3. For example, in the case R. v. Aaron Caffrey (Southwark Crown Court, 17 October 2003), Caffrey's defence presumably convinced a jury that Caffrey did not launch the attacks against the Port of Houston himself, and that hackers carried out the attacks using a Trojan they had placed in Caffrey's computer.

More recently however, in 2005, although the court initially upheld the view that such a DoS attack would not be an offence under s 3, this decision was overturned on appeal and the defendant, Lennon, was subsequently convicted (DPP v. Lennon [2006] EWHC 1201). He had sent 5 million emails to his ex-employer, causing the email server to fail. It is probably no coincidence that prior to the decision being reached on appeal, the CMA had been reworded within the Police and Justice Bill 2006, clarifying that DoS attacks certainly constitute an offence under the revised s 3 of the CMA.

The new s 3(1) no longer includes the term 'modification' and refers instead to an 'act' in relation to a computer. The new s 3(3) also refers to reckless acts; it is no longer necessary to prove intent. This broadens the scope of the Act, and in addition, penalties for s 3 offences have also been increased. A new section (s 3A) is also to be introduced. The new s3 (subsections 1 to 5 inclusive) reads as follows:

> Unauthorised acts with intent to impair, or with recklessness as to impairing, operation of computer, etc.

1. A person is guilty of an offence if:

    (a) he does any unauthorised act in relation to a computer;

    (b) at the time when he does the act he knows that it is unauthorised; and

    (c) either subsection (2) or subsection (3) below applies.

2. This subsection applies if the person intends by doing the act:

    (a) to impair the operation of any computer,

    (b) to prevent or hinder access to any program or data held in any computer,

    (c) to impair the operation of any such program or the reliability of any such data,

3. This subsection applies if the person is reckless as to whether the act will do any of the things mentioned in paragraphs (a) to (d) of subsection (2) above.

4. The intention referred to in subsection (2) above, or the recklessness referred to in subsection (3) above, need not relate to:

    (a) any particular computer;

(b) any particular program or data; or

(c) a program or data of any particular kind.

5. In this section:

    (a) a reference to doing an act includes a reference to causing an act to be done;

    (b) 'act' includes a series of acts;

    (c) a reference to impairing, preventing or hindering something includes a reference to doing so temporarily.

Section 37 of the Police & Justice Act 2006 will also create a new offence, (inserted after s 3 of the CMA):

    S.3A Making, supplying or obtaining articles for use in offence under section 1 or 3

1. A person is guilty of an offence if he makes, adapts, supplies or offers to supply any article intending it to be used to commit, or to assist in the commission of, an offence under section 1 or 3.

2. A person is guilty of an offence if he supplies or offers to supply any article believing that it is likely to be used to commit, or to assist in the commission of, an offence under section 1 or 3.

3. A person is guilty of an offence if he obtains any article with a view to its being supplied for use to commit, or to assist in the commission of, an offence under section 1 or 3.

4. In this section 'article' includes any program or data held in electronic form.

Note however that an offence will not have been committed under s 3A unless every act or other event (proof of which is required for conviction of that offence) takes place after s 37 of the Police & Justice Act 2006 comes into force.

2.2.2 Other recent changes to legislation

Apart from changes to the CMA 1990, other pieces of legislation have been amended in response to problematic activities involving new communication and information technologies.

In 2005, Straszkiewicz was prosecuted (Watts, 2005) for the unauthorised use of a domestic wireless network, an offence under s 125 and 126 of the Communications Act 2003. (The use of such a network would not have been an offence under the CMA unless there had been unauthorised access or unauthorised modification to the computer as well.) The suspect was caught standing outside a dwelling in a residential area using a wireless enabled laptop. He was found guilty of 'dishonestly obtaining an electronic communications service and possessing equipment for fraudulent use of a communications service'. The Crown Prosecution Service confirmed he was 'piggybacking' the wireless network of private households.

Worthy of specific mention within this chapter is The Fraud Act 2006, as it is the most recently enacted piece of legislation that specifically impacts digital crime. Prior to the implementation of the Fraud Act 2006 a deception must have worked on a mind; a person had to be deceived. This caused difficulties for investigators of fraud involving technology; it was often a machine that had been deceived, and in terms of pre-2006 law a machine could not be deceived. For example, in the case R. v. Moritz (Acton Crown Court, 19 June 1981 (unreported)) the court heard that false VAT returns had been filed, but they were read only by a computer; it was held that there was no evidence of deception as Customs and Excise were unable to prove that any personnel had been deceived, since the returns were dealt with in a fully automated way. The definition of deception clearly required modification.

Further difficulties arising from the definition of deception followed, and in 2002 the Law Commission issued a consultation paper followed by a report. This recommended that offences of deception under the Theft Acts 1968–1996 should be repealed, and that the common law crime of 'conspiracy to defraud' should be abolished. Two new statutory offences were proposed: fraud and obtaining services dishonestly. There can be no doubt that Article 8 of the Council of Europe Convention on Cybercrime influenced these proposals; the Article, to be implemented in the near future, states that:

> Each party shall adopt such legislative and other measures as may be necessary to establish as criminal offences under its domestic law,

when committed intentionally and without right, the causing of loss of property to another by:

(a) any input, alteration, deletion or suppression of computer data,

(b) any interference with the functioning of a computer system,

with fraudulent or dishonest intent of procuring, without right, an economic benefit for oneself or for another.

The Fraud Act 2006 came into force in January 2007 and created a new general offence of fraud (s 1) with a maximum sentence of 10 years, replacing all previous deception offences. Sections 2, 3 and 4 introduce three possible ways of committing fraud and list the associated offences. However, despite the recommendation, the common law offence of conspiracy to defraud has not been abolished.

Section 2 of the Fraud Act 2006 makes it an offence to commit fraud by false representation. The representation must be made dishonestly, with the intention of making a gain or causing a loss (or a risk of loss to another person), but the gain or loss does not have to actually take place. The representation may be expressed or implied, and can be stated in words or communicated by conduct. There is no limitation on the way in which the representation may be expressed, so it could be written, spoken or posted on a web site. It could also be expressed by way of conduct, for example the dishonest use of a credit card to pay for items. The offence would also be committed by someone who engages in phishing. Subsection 2(5) provides that a representation be regarded as made if it is submitted:

- in any form;
- to any system or device designed to receive communications; or
- with or without human intervention.

Note the care with which this legislation has been worded; it is difficult to conceive of a form of representation that would not be covered.

Section 3 of the Fraud Act 2006 makes it an offence to commit fraud by failing to disclose information to another person where there is a legal duty to disclose the information. An example could be a holidaymaker who does not disclose requested medical information when applying for travel insurance.

Section 4 of the Fraud Act 2006 makes it an offence to commit a fraud by dishonestly abusing one's position. It applies in situations where the defendant has been put in a privileged position, and by virtue of this position is expected to safeguard other people's financial interests, or not to act against those interests. This Act has removed the need to prove that the mind of a person has been deceived in order to complete the offence, and indeed the legislators (within the explanatory notes of the Act) give specific examples in respect of phishing, website postings and so on.

As well as the Fraud Act 2006, other legislative changes have been made in order to broaden the concept of deception. The VAT Act 1994 has been amended to read 'deception includes deceiving a machine', and certain sections of road traffic legislation have also been rewritten; it is now possible in law to deceive a parking meter.

2.2.3 Proposed changes to legislation

As well as the proposed amendments to the CMA discussed above, proposed changes to other areas of legislation are likely to impact on digital crime and subsequent prosecutions. These proposals are included within the Criminal Justice and Immigration Bill, which received its first reading in June 2007.

At present, simple possession of obscene material is not an offence under the Obscene Publications Act 1959, although under s 2 of the Act it is an offence to publish an obscene article (whether for gain or not), or to possess an obscene article for publication for gain. Therefore, the present Act would not cover someone downloading material from the internet purely for their own use, however extreme the material. However, in August 2006 the Home Office announced that under s 64 of the Criminal Justice and Immigration Bill, simple possession of violent and extreme pornographic material will become a criminal offence punishable by up to 3 years imprisonment. The type of material to be covered would be of the same nature as that covered under s 2 of the Obscene Publications Act 1959. The new law is intended to ensure possession of violent and extreme pornography is illegal both on and offline. Section 70 of the Criminal Justice and Immigration Bill also increases the penalty for the offences linked to the publication of obscene articles from 3 years to a maximum of 5 years imprisonment.

The same Bill also contains proposed amendments to the Indecent Images of Children Act 1978. At the present time, offences under this Act relate to indecent photographs and pseudo-photographs, including video recordings and images held on computers or the internet. Pseudo-photographs also include computer generated images, and a pseudo-photograph will be considered as being that of a child even if some of its characteristics are those of an adult. Section 68 of the Bill expands the definition of a photograph to include any images derived from photographs or pseudo photographs. Such images would include a tracing or other image (whether made by electronic or other means) which is not itself a photograph or pseudo-photograph, but which is derived from the whole or part of a photograph or pseudo-photograph. It will also include data stored on a computer disk (or by other electronic means) which is capable of conversion into an image. These proposed amendments aim to close some of the potential 'loopholes' within the current definition of a photograph; new loopholes brought about by new techniques for generating images.

Pseudo-photographs and non-photographic visual depictions of child sexual abuse

Robin Bryant

It is has been an offence, for a number of years (under the Protection of Children Act 1978 and the Criminal Justice Act 1988) to possess indecent photographs and pseudo-photographs of children.

Pseudo-photographs are defined by section 7 of the Protection of Children Act 1978 (as amended by the Criminal Justice and Public Order Act 1994) as an image, whether made by computer-graphics or otherwise howsoever, which appears to be a photograph.

Further, the Act explains that if the impression conveyed by a pseudo-photograph is that the person shown is a child, the pseudo-photograph shall be treated for all purposes as showing a child, and so shall a pseudo-photograph where the predominant impression conveyed is that the person shown is a child (notwithstanding that some of the physical characteristics shown are those of an adult).

References in the law to an indecent pseudo-photograph are also taken to include:

(a) a copy of an indecent pseudo-photograph; and

(b) data stored on a computer disc or by other electronic means which is capable of conversion into a pseudo-photograph.

Under the new Criminal Justice and Immigration Bill it is proposed that it will also become an offence to possess non-photographic visual depictions of child sexual abuse. This will cover visual depictions such as Computer Generated Images (CGIs; for example animated imagery), cartoons (for example, 'Manga' type) and other forms of fantasy-style imagery. These types of depictions might potentially be used for grooming purposes.

Under the proposed new legislation possession of visual depictions containing content in one or more of the following areas would be an offence:

- non-penetrative sexual activity between adults and children;

- penetrative sexual activity involving a child or children, or between children and adults;

- sadism or bestiality involving a child.

The NSPCC cites evidence that non-photographic visual images are being encountered 'more frequently in the possession of persons being arrested for or being charged with child pornography offences' (NSPCC, 2007, p. 1). In some cases non-photographic visual depictions may have been derived electronically from photographic originals: whereas possession of the original would be an offence, possession of the derivative is not yet so.

For further reading on this subject, full details of the Acts referred to within this text are available from the Office of Public Sector Information at www.opsi.gov.uk. Updates in respect of progress of the Bills mentioned can be obtained via www.parliament.uk.

Questions

Robin Bryant & Sarah Bryant

1. Approximately what proportion of EU nations have ratified the Convention on Cybercrime at the present time (2007)?

2. What is the key aim of the European Commission's 'Proposal for a Council Framework Decision on attacks against information systems'?

3. How are EC directives relevant to countering digital crime (e.g. the Electronic Commerce (EC Directive) Regulations 2002) enacted within UK law?

4. Which section of the CMA 1990 relates to 'Unauthorised access with intent to commit or facilitate the commission of a further offence'?

5. Why is PACE 1984 of relevance to a digital crime investigator?

6. What particular difficulties are likely to be encountered in a prosecution for a hacking offence under the 1971 Criminal Damage Act?

7. Which 2006 Act contains important amendments to the CMA 1990?

References

Council of Europe (2001) Convention on Cybercrime, Budapest, 23.XI.2001.[Online]. Available at: http://conventions.coe.int/Treaty/en/Treaties/Html/185.htm (Accessed: Oct 9 2007).

Grabosky, P. and Smith, R. (2001) Telecommunications fraud in the digital age: the convergence of technologies. In: Wall, D. (ed.) *Crime and the Internet*. London: Routledge.

Hansard (Commons) April 5 2005, column 1293 [Online]. Available at: http://www.publications.parliament.uk/pa/cm200405/cmhansrd/vo050405/debtext/50405-15.htm (Accessed: Oct 9 2007).

NSPCC (2007) *The CHIS coalition response to the consultation on the possession of non-photographic visual depictions of child sexual abuse*. [Online]. Available at: http://www.nspcc.org.uk/Inform/policyandpublicaffairs/Consultations/2007/2007_CHIS_nonphotographic_images_wdf48632.pdf (Accessed: Oct 15 2007).

Watts, A. (2005) Court cracks down on dishonest Wi-Fi user. [Online]. Available at: http://www.abcmoney.co.uk/news/272005548.htm (Accessed: Oct 9 2007).

3

Investigating Digital Crime

Ian Kennedy

Digital forensics is a relatively recent addition to the forensics family and, for this reason alone, the terminology used is undergoing constant definition and redefinition. An increasing number of books are available with titles that make reference to terms such as 'cyberforensics', 'computer forensics', 'Windows forensics' and 'Intrusion forensics'. As we shall see throughout this chapter, not only is the terminology in a state of development but the training and accreditation is changing too.

Hi-tech crime is often associated with computers and especially with the investigation of paedophiles. Whilst this may reflect the current caseload of many law enforcement high tech (or hi-tech) crime units around the UK, it is becoming increasingly common for digital devices other than personal computers to be either the target of a crime, or to be used to assist in the commission of a crime. Mobile phones, digital cameras, personal data assistants (PDAs), mp3 players, and even online storage are currently the technologies of choice for the technically savvy criminal. Digital forensics therefore, extends beyond the confines of the computer and encompasses a broad range of digital technology.

Investigating Digital Crime   Edited by Robin Bryant and Sarah Bryant
© 2008 John Wiley & Sons, Ltd

Evidence and intelligence in digital crime

Robin Bryant

Evidence and intelligence are both forms of information that may be used in an enquiry and a subsequent prosecution.

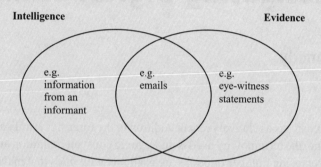

Figure 3.1 Intelligence and evidence

Intelligence is information which, when analysed and interpreted, is of potential value in progressing an enquiry into an alleged, suspected or actual crime. Information from a paid informant for example might constitute intelligence. Evidence, in comparison, is any information which may be of value to a court in deciding on the issues presented to them, most fundamentally on the guilt or innocence of the accused. For a digital crime, recovered parts of an email communication might constitute intelligence and evidence. Not all intelligence will be used as evidence (for example, a recovered deleted SMS communication may suggest a certain line of enquiry), and not all evidence is intelligence (for example, a statement that a witness makes in court). Legislation in the UK governing the collection of intelligence and evidence is extensive.

There are many potential sources of digital crime evidence and intelligence, and some are shown in tables 3.1 and 3.2 below. One unusual requirement for the work of a forensic digital investigator is a broad familiarity with technology, both ancient and modern. For example it is perfectly feasible that a criminal has continued to use his or her reliable Amstrad PCW word-processor to this day. For this reason, police high tech crime units sometimes include impressive repositories of knowledge about defunct computer and word processing equipment. Many types of office and domestic electrical equipment contain digital memory, and at least some may provide intelligence or even evidence to support an investigation. The list in table 3.1 (below) reflects the wide range of equipment that may be used by offenders.

Table 3.1 Sources of digital information

Sources	Examples
Hard drives	'Winchester' drives, tape drives, IDE drives (2.5 inch, 3.5 inch, 5.25 inch), SCSI drives, ATA drives, DMA drives and external drives.
Discs, tapes, cartridges and pens	Floppy discs (relatively common 3.5in, less common 4.5in, 5.25in); Zip drive cartridges; Jaz drive cartridges; tapes for external tape drives; CD (including miniCD); DVD (including miniDVD, HDDVD, Blu-ray); USB flashdrives (pens or memory sticks).
Network devices, modems and routers	Servers; Network Interface (NIC) cards; internal, external, PCMIA card modems; routers (including wireless routers). Also included under this heading would be the associated software e.g. the configuration file for a home modem/router.
Memory cards	Used in a variety of devices, including digital cameras and laptops. Memory cards include Memory Sticks, Multimedia Cards (MMC), CompactFlash (CF), SmartMedia and Secure Digital (SD, miniSD).
Computer access control devices	These devices include stripe (swipe) cards, dongles, smartcards, keycards, fingerprint recognition pads. Most are a combination of hardware with software. These devices may elicit information concerning the users of the devices.
Volatile memory	Dumped RAM (including passwords and passphrases), state of open network connections.
Personal media players	Included here are 'Walkmans' (cassette, minidisc and CD), mp3 players, multimedia players (e.g. an Archos). Some of these devices (such as an mp3 player) can also save non-music data such as image files.
Recording machines (sound)	Tape machines include: • reel-to-reel tape machines; • cassette recorders players (tapes in C30, C45 and C60 sizes); • answer machines (smaller tape cassettes); • hand held recorders. Some of these machines may have been used to record data (e.g. from a Sinclair Spectrum). CD players/recorders.

Table 3.1   (*Continued*)

Sources	Examples
Digital cameras and camcorders	As well as the images themselves (with date stamps etc.), digital camera memory is also normally able to store other forms of data.
Recording machines (linked to TVs)	VHS video players/recorders. DVD players/recorders (a DVD player may be used to show digital photographs from a USB pen).
Mobile phones, electronic organisers, PDAs and smart devices	Including numerous mobile phone makes; Psion, iPAQ, Apple Newton, Palm Pilot, Blackberry, Trio and i-phone. Pagers, although no longer used by the public in the UK, might still contain useful contact information.
GPS devices	Including GPS devices within cars and hand-held devices (including within mobile phones).
Office equipment	'Telex' machines, fax machines, scanners, printers, photocopiers may all have residual memory information.
Games consoles	NES, SNES, Playstation etc. For example a 'chipped' Microsoft Xbox may have been set up as an ftp server, or a games console may have been used to take part in a chat room.
TV and radio	Digital TVs, digital satellite TV receivers, digital radios
White goods	Microwave cookers and washing machines.
Others	Digital clocks and watches.

3.1 Digital evidence

Quite apart from the legal position on digital evidence, conveying the significance of the evidence itself to the court presents a particular challenge. It is not enough to simply translate technical data into layman's terms as one might translate a foreign language into English. The technical complexity of such cases frequently surpasses the technical knowledge and experience of the court. Some items of evidence may simply seem intangible to a court due to their 'virtual' nature or their confusing similarity to other items of evidence. For example, consider trying to explain the difference between the last access date and the last modified date on an NTFS file system.

Thus, unlike a written document, raw computer evidence must be presented alongside an accurate interpretation which clearly identifies its significance in the context of where it was found. For example, the hard disk of a computer contains raw binary data, and ignoring more complex data types, this may be encoded as simple binary, binary coded decimal or as hexadecimal data. The value encoded may represent a numeric, alphanumeric, date/time or logical value. Even dates and times can be encoded in a number of ways employing, for example, a 'big endian' or 'little endian' approach in terms of representation.

The interpretation of evidence must be undertaken by a suitably qualified person and then presented in an accessible form for perusal by a court. Over simplification is dangerous as it could lead to the data becoming open to interpretation. Any doubt as to the interpretation of a single item of evidence can often be addressed by correlating it with other evidence such as log files, internet history, and link files.

Unlike some conventional crime scenes, the very existence of evidence may not be obvious to the 'first responder' (the first person to arrive) at a digital crime scene. It is not likely that there will be easily identifiable items of evidence such as footprints or bloodstains to be identified and preserved. Conventional forensics follows the ethos of Locard's exchange principle as described by Thornton (1997); namely 'Every contact leaves a trace'. Akin to evidence such as DNA, digital evidence is also fragile and easily contaminated or damaged. Every click of the mouse could potentially alter data stored on a device and thus destroy vital evidence. Thus, a first responder must not switch on a computer, or 'have a look around' on a machine that is already running, as this threatens the integrity of the evidence contained on the computer. Such integrity was debased recently (BBC, 2007g) by a Special Branch detective who breached standard police procedure when he switched on a laptop computer and explored its contents (for over an hour) prior to passing it over to a forensic computer analyst for examination.

Digital forensic investigation in context

Robin Bryant

For a digital forensic investigation to be successful, several different perspectives need to be taken into account, and the three most important considerations are shown in figure 3.2.

For example, examining the image of a SIM card from a mobile phone cannot be regarded as simply a scientific process (the Scientific Disciplines perspective). The examination is taking place because of an investigation (the Law Enforcement perspective) with all that follows from this; possibly in order to corroborate an account for the purpose of furthering an enquiry.

For the enquiry to lead to a successful prosecution, the perspective of the Criminal Justice System (and in particular, the CPS) must also be considered e.g. ACPO principles must have been adhered to, particularly in relation to evidential requirements.

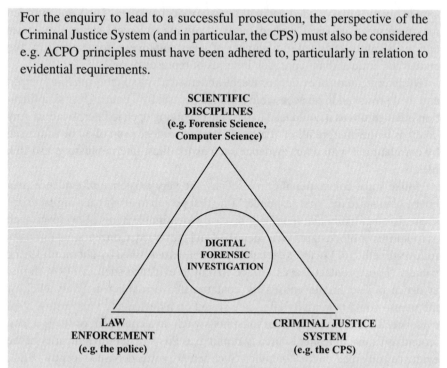

Figure 3.2   Factors impinging on a digital forensic investigation

3.2 How a digital device becomes involved in a crime

Although many crimes committed with the use of a computer may seem to be quite modern, they often include a number of features that may be somewhat more traditional in nature. Using eBay, for example, to offer goods for sale, receive payment and then fail to supply the goods to the customer is essentially a traditional fraud; an old crime committed using a high tech method. Aspects of the same offence can be committed using a newspaper advert or even a handshake with an exchange of cash in the local pub. It is debated elsewhere in this book just how 'new' these forms of criminality really are.

Not all crimes committed using a digital device use it simply as a means to an end. A denial of service (DoS) attack on a website, or the intentional distribution of a virus designed to manipulate data stored on a victim's computer are both examples of crimes in which the computer itself is the target of the crime; the computer has not simply been used in the commission of the offence.

There are numerous ways in which a digital device may feature within a crime. Some particular examples are discussed in this section.

3.2.1 Fraud and identity theft

The Advance Fee or '419' fraud is a popular confidence trick frequently perpetrated by West African organised crime networks. The 419 reference is taken from the section of the Nigerian Criminal Code relating to Fraud (International Centre for Nigerian Law, 2007). It is a particularly old form of attempted fraud that dates back to the 16th century when it was known as the 'Spanish Prisoner' scam, but its commission is most certainly facilitated through the use of digital technology. Put simply, the scam involves a victim being offered a large sum of money, but in order to access this money the victim must pay a fee in advance. The reasons cited for this are varied but one example is to pay some form of tax to an organisation holding the money. Further requests for payment are then subsequently made until the victim realises what is happening at which point the scammer stops all correspondence and disappears. Figure 3.3 shows a more subtle variant of this scam; a request for money is likely to follow shortly!

Phishing is another modern twist on an old crime. Contacting victims electronically via email, the scammers use social engineering techniques, and masquerade as a legitimate organisation. The organisations of choice are currently eBay, PayPal and certain high street banks. In a recent high profile attack the website Monster.com had a number of its recruiter accounts compromised, and these accounts were then used to log in and obtain the personal details of candidates. Candidate data was then uploaded to a remote server whcih eventually held over 1.6 million entries (Symantec Corporation, 2007a) containing personal information belonging to several hundred thousand candidates, mainly based in the US, who had posted their résumés to the Monster.com website.

Typically, the potential phishing victim is sent an email purportedly from the legitimate organisation with a link to its website that, when visited, superficially looks genuine. The victim is then asked to log in to 'verify' their security details. In some cases additional details such as credit card and corresponding PIN numbers are also requested. Manipulating people into divulging confidential information in this way is more of a problem than one might presume. Dhamija *et al.* (2006) recently completed a study that showed 40 per cent of a test group failed to spot phishing sites while the most sophisticated site fooled 90 per cent of the group.

Hello, dear friend!

My name is Ekaterina. I am 26 years old. I'm from Russia, city Cheboksary.
I live together with my mum and I work as adviser on sale home appliances.
I have many various hobbies: sport, a photo, drawing. I dream to have strong and happy family.
It's my purpose in life. I want to be happy and to do happy my family.
Recently I thought that I have it already. However.......
I wish to tell you history which have pushed me write to you.
6-7 months ago I have got acquainted with man from your country.
His name is Peter. Our meeting was at a seminar in city St.Peterburg.
It was the working meeting. Between us began the novel.
It was so fast and I thought that it's my man. Through 3 days he has left
home. We have understood that letters can not replace our meeting face to face again.
Peter has told that I should arrive to him!!! I was very glad during that moment. I wrote the application for reception visa. I
waited reception = visa approximately half of year.
All this time Peter called and wrote to me letters. All things was very good. I have received the invitation from the ambassador for
reception =sa. My director has given me holiday from work and I have gone to Moscow to receive visa.
I said this good news to Peter, but he told that he does not want our meeting. He played with me. He has told me that he has wife
with 3!!!! children and now he don't want our meeting. I have been broken...
I could not think that it was game with my feelings..... I did not think that people are so severe......
Now I am in Moscow and waiting for reception visa.
I don't want that all was gone for nothing and will be glad if my visa will be useful to our meeting.
I could arrive already in 7-8 days, but I have problem. I don't know any man who would like my arrival.
I hope that it will not sound silly if I will ask you about our meeting and good time together...
I don't know your ideas about my letter, but it would be fine if we could meet and have some weeks or months together.
I want to use my visa for trip to your country and search man with which I would like to have happy and strong family.
I was never married and have no any children. I'm woman which ready to creation family with good man.
I don't know about you anything, but I want it very much.
It would be fine if we could meet, to do friendship or more than simply friendship.
I will be happy if you also have a free time and we could meet soon.
I don't know about your plans at present time, but I sincerely hope that we can have meeting with you in the near future.
You can write all that you want. Ask any questions which interest you.
I hope that you understand my English I began to study English approximately 1,5 year ago. Write to me back and I will tell more
about myself and send my photos.

Please, write to me back and send your photos on my regular e-mail: katykitten@bk.ru

Have a good day,
Ekaterina

Figure 3.3 A variant of the 419 scam

As noted in an earlier chapter of this book, the recently updated Fraud Act 2006 includes an amendment to Section 2, fraud by false representation. The Explanatory Notes (Great Britain. Office of Public Sector Information, 2006) state that anyone engaging in the act of phishing is guilty of fraud by false representation.

Using phishing techniques to obtain confidential information has recently led to a number of cases of identity theft. This is the practice of using personal details from another person to open bank accounts, and obtain credit cards, loans, state benefits and documents such as passports and driving licences in a victim's name.

Recent cases include a woman who impersonated her sister's identity to obtain a mortgage (BBC, 2007f), a university tutor who stole nearly £20 000 on two credit cards he had taken out in the name of his former landlords (BBC, 2007h) and a man who headed a £2.3m identity theft ring targeting the bank accounts of a vicar, businessmen and even the dead (BBC, 2007b). Garlik (2007) recently published a report indicating that during 2006 there were 92 000 cases of reported online identity theft and, it was claimed that 40 per cent of these were committed online. A recent report by security firm Symantec (2007b) indicated that its software alone had been used to block 12.5 million phishing emails per day over the first six months of 2007.

3.2.2 Computer misuse

For computer misuse offences, both the offence and the method used to commission the offence involve computers. The Computer Misuse Act 1990 was established to legislate against offenders who gain unauthorised access to computer systems, possibly with intent to commit further offences or modify any data contained on the target computer system. This is discussed in more detail in Chapter 2.

Computer misuse offences include:

- accessing areas of a competitor's website without authorisation and downloading a large amount of internal information;

- sending a large number (millions) of emails to a former employer's email server causing a system crash, known as a Denial of Service or 'DoS' attack;

- writing and distributing computer viruses and inciting others to spread computer viruses.

There were 144 500 reported cases of computer misuse (excluding malware) alone during 2006, and it has been estimated that over 6 000 000 unreported malware incidents are likely to have occurred in the same year (Garlik, 2007) Malware is discussed in more detail in Chapter 4.

Another area of emerging computer crime is that of an offender connecting to a victim's Wi-fi connection without permission. A recent case reported by the BBC (2007d) highlights that such dishonesty in obtaining free internet access is an offence under the Communications Act 2003 and a potential breach of the Computer Misuse Act 1990. This type of activity is discussed in more detail in Chapter 8.

3.2.3 Sexual offences

It has been estimated that some 850 000 sexual approaches are likely to have been made to children over the internet during 2006 (Garlik, 2007). Such offences are found to occur primarily as a result of an offender visiting searching and/or browsing websites, newsgroups or peer to peer networks. The receipt (and in some cases distribution) of email and media such as CD-ROMs may also constitute an offence. In some cases webcam technology has been used in combination with grooming to make an indecent image of a child.

Grooming is the act of an adult communicating with a child with the intention of meeting with the child to commit a further, often sexual, offence. O'Connell (2007) identifies five stages of the grooming process:

1. *Friendship*. In this initial stage flattery is used by the adult to encourage the child into talking in a private chatroom where they will be isolated. It is common for a non-sexual picture of the child to be requested.

2. *Forming a relationship*. The child is asked what problems they have. This creates the illusion of the adult being their best friend.

3. *Risk assessment*. To assess the risk of being detected the adult will at this stage often ask the child about the location of their computer and who else has access to it.

4. *Exclusivity*. With the friendship and risk level established, the groomer then embarks on a process of building up a sense of mutual love and trust with the child. A sense of complete non-judgemental friendship is established, giving the child the feeling they can discuss 'anything'.

5. *Sex talk*. In the final stage, explicit conversations are initiated with the child. Frequently too, the child is asked to supply sexually explicit pictures of themselves. At this stage too, the paedophile will usually try to arrange a meeting with the child.

The offender has a wide range of choice; the means of performing this type of offence are rich and varied. Conventional chat sessions such as MSN and Yahoo Messenger (with or without the use of a webcam) are relatively simple to set up as no 'profile' is required to initiate a chat session. Social networking websites such as www.bebo.com and www.facebook.com generally require the user to create a profile before initiating contact with other users, but the details required for the profile are usually minimal and easily falsified. The sense of anonymity often experienced by offenders using the internet gives them the confidence to perform actions that they might consider unthinkable in real world. These issues are explored in more detail in Chapter 10.

3.2.4 Mobile phones

Recent advances in mobile phone technology have created mobile phones that include a digital camera. Increased memory capacity, removable memory cards, higher still picture resolution and the ability to store several minutes of video footage inevitably make the mobile phone an attractive and portable option for many people, a few of whom will choose to use it to commit offences.

Guardian news and Media Limited (2007) report a number of teenagers arrested for example, for using mobile phones to take indecent images of other children. The BBC (2007a) reports that a barrister too has fallen foul of this technology by allegedly using a mobile phone camera to take covert pictures of girls on trains.

The act of 'happy slapping' is another example of a modern twist on an old crime, reports Guardian news and Media Limited (2005). This is the act of committing an assault or robbery while an accomplice records the act, often with a mobile phone. Sexual assaults (BBC, 2007e) and even murder (BBC, 2007c) have also been recorded in this manner.

3.3 Forensic examination in practice

The precise procedure used for the examination of a digital device is of vital importance. Aside from the accreditation issues discussed later, there are no nationally agreed standards, rules or protocol for the handling of computer evidence. There are certainly ACPO guidelines for the handling of such evidence, but they are little more than best practice advice.

From a prosecution point of view a forensic examination of a digital device is generally considered to be conducted in four primary stages:

- acquisition;
- identification;
- evaluation; and
- presentation.

The acquisition stage is concerned with the forensically sound capture of the data. A digital device involved in a crime is effectively a crime scene in its own right which needs to be secured, just as much as a murder scene. Like fingerprint and DNA evidence, digital evidence is fragile and easily lost if appropriate precautions are not followed. Horror stories of over-zealous police officers switching on digital cameras to look for evidence or conducting virus scans on floppy disks prior to submitting them for a forensic examination still haunt investigators working in the field. The location in which the exhibit was found and seized is also an important factor to record as it can reveal a great deal about the intent of the suspected offender. For example, was the wireless device hidden beneath floorboards, or was it in an open access area like a living room?

One of the most important aspects of the acquisition stage is the process of forensically copying the data from the digital device onto an 'evidence disk'. The accepted best practice to achieve this is to use a hardware write-blocking device. The device is installed between the evidence disk and the forensic workstation, and only allows data to pass in one direction. It is designed to stop any write signals being passed from the receiving computer back to the evidence disk, hence preserving the data contained on the evidence disk in its original form.

Data recovery from hard drives

Robin Bryant

Digital forensic investigation frequently involves the recovery of digital information from PCs, PDAs, mobile phones, GPS devices and indeed just about any device with electronic memory. Some of these may contain memory in the form of a hard drive and the device may also employ a Windows GUI interface. In terms of digital forensics, files and folders on a hard drive can be thought of as falling into one of four different categories (our terminology):

'Obvious' These are files and folders which are obviously either part of the operating system (e.g. MS Word), or files (such as an MS Word document) which have been saved by a particular program. Some of these are certainly of potential interest to the digital forensic investigator. For example, one useful folder in Windows XP might be found in the folder C:\Documents and Settings\User\Local Settings\Temporary Internet Files. This folder contains information concerning internet sites visited with dates and times.

'Obscure' These are files and folders which, although not necessarily hidden (by the user or by the default setting of the GUI), do not have an obvious meaning or use. Examples include 'temp' files which may have the format '*.tmp' where * is a wildcard (e.g. ~WRL0554.tmp). For example, when using MS Word, copies of the document are often saved as *.tmp files which can usually be read as a document, by either changing the file extension to 'doc' or by associating MS Word with the file extension. (Although, in practice, an alternative program to the original would probably be used in a forensic investigation to examine the file, in order to avoid modifying the original.)

'Hidden' These are files and folders which, although still present and intact on the hard drive, are hidden from the user. They will not even be revealed by ticking the 'Show hidden files and folders' checkbox within the normal Windows routine.

'Deleted' These are files which have either been deliberately deleted by the user (for example, in Windows, by sending a file to the 'Recycle Bin' and then emptying the bin) or have been automatically deleted, perhaps on booting up. A fundamental premise of the forensic recovery of deleted data is that it is actually surprisingly difficult for a person to completely and irretrievably delete a file. Unless special software is used, or particular command line actions taken, the likelihood is that at least part of the deleted file is actually still present on the hard drive (particularly with more modern PCs with large capacity hard drives).

However, note that there are also other 'file residues' that may be located, such as ambient data, file slack, free space, and shadow data. The 'page file' is possibly the most important type of ambient data. Page files are found with all Windows operating systems as a form of electronic 'scratch pad' to write data when additional random access memory is needed and may contain logon names, passwords and fragments of messages and documents. Most users are unaware of the existence of the page file. Other areas containing file or folder details include registry, thumb.db files, email attachments and event logs.

The recovery of obscure, hidden and deleted files is usually one of the tasks of a digital forensic investigator. As an example consider the forensics of retrieving information concerning a person's use of the internet from an image of their PC's hard drive. Apart from examining obvious and obscure files and folders and attempting the recovery of deleted files, the investigator would also probably access a hidden folder called 'content.ie5' which contains a file called 'index.dat'. This file records information about any websites visited, and (unusually) is not deleted by clearing the temporary internet files from folders. The content of the .ie5 folder and index.dat file will not be made visible using the usual Windows 'Show hidden files and folders' tab. It will be made visible however, by running the command <dir/ a "%Userprofile%\Local Settings\Temporary Internet Files*.*" >. (Dedicated forensically validated software is commercially available for this procedure, and in addition provides a user-friendly interface for collecting the information).

In the identification stage, the precise location of relevant digital data must be established. A computer with two hard disks, for example, can be initially considered at a physical level in terms of a base unit, disk 1 and disk 2. Examples of the properties that are of interest from this perspective are the system date and time on the base unit, the number of sectors on both disks and whether any hidden sectors reside on either disk. At a logical level, the number and type of partitions present, and the type and structure of the file system are also of interest; they may reveal much about the owner's level of knowledge. Finally, the identification stage considers the context within which any evidence is found. A good example of this is when a particular credit card number (significant within an investigation) is found in the area of a hard disk where previous files once resided, known as unallocated clusters. Here, ghosts of former files reside in part or even in full and these may be used to identify the original context of the credit card number; for instance, was the card number in the content of an email? This may be crucial if the evidence is to be exhibited for use in court.

In the evaluation stage a decision on the relevance of the find is made. A clear understanding is required of how the data was produced, when it was produced and by whom. It is at this stage that the common defence of Trojans and pop-ups in internet browsing-related offences can be discounted through the examination of any malware found on the device, live port activity and internet searching habits, for example.

The presentation stage involves the interpretation of the raw data and the reconstruction of events that occurred on the exhibit prior to its seizure. The report must be technically concise, but clearly written for the lay person if it is to be understood by the court. The author of the report must be prepared to be questioned and perhaps even defend their findings in a court of law.

3.3.1 Best practice principles

ACPO have published the *Good Practice Guide* for the recovery of computer-based electronic evidence (Association of Chief Police Officers of England, 2007). In this document they identify four primary guidelines, which we summarise here:

Principle 1: no action taken should change data held on an exhibit.

Principle 2: where a person finds it necessary to access original data held on an exhibit that person must be competent to do so and be able to give evidence explaining the relevance and the implications of their actions.

Principle 3: an audit trail of all processes applied to an exhibit should be created and preserved. This should be repeatable to an independent third party.

Principle 4: the person in charge of the investigation (the case officer) has overall responsibility for ensuring that the law and these principles are adhered to.

These principles influence many of the procedures followed when examining a digital device. Thus, the acquisition stage must preserve and not alter the state of the exhibit and thereby uphold Principle 1. Under certain circumstances, such as when acquiring data from a corporate server, it is impractical to take the device offline and so data from selected areas of the server must be captured. (Other areas of the server may be inaccessible to the suspect, so are not required for the investigation.) To adhere to Principle 2, the impact of these actions must be known and should only be undertaken by a competent person. When identifying and evaluating evidence a comprehensive set of contemporaneous notes must be made in order to record and document the processing of an exhibit, in accordance with Principle 3.

3.4 Professional accreditation

Digital forensics is a new and developing field, and is increasingly recognised as a scientific discipline in its own right. More and more organisations are offering services, seminars, courses and accreditation in an effort to define and become the *de facto* standard in this specialised market.

This open market approach has led to a number of problems for managers of forensic units and staff, particularly within the court system of England and Wales. First, there is no single and mandatory regulatory body to provide a line of professional accountability for digital forensics specialists. Professional accountability is of vital importance for practitioners, particularly when liaising with other professionals and institutions. Practising lawyers, for example, are answerable to the Bar Standards Board and medical doctors are answerable to the British Medical Association (BMA).

Second, there is no digital forensics professional qualification that is universally recognised as the professional standard. For example, professional engineers are frequently expected to possess Chartered Engineer (CEng) status; this is a recognised standard for engineering, but for digital forensics there are at present two registers (and both are optional), one within the Council for the Registration of Forensic Practitioners and the other being developed by Skills for Justice.

There is also no single nationwide training programme for digital forensics specialists. The implications of this are significant. First, there is no nationally agreed career path for a digital forensic examiner, and therefore no way of establishing that an individual is 'qualified' to practise. Second, there is no 'best practice' or industry standard on how to undertake the various processes used to analyse digital data.

Currently, it is left very much up to the court to accept the credentials and experience of an individual prior to accepting their evidence in court. This can and does lead to a forensic examiner's credibility being challenged in an attempt to have their testimony rejected by the court. The primary cause of this situation is the infancy of the field. From a law enforcement perspective, investigations involving the forensic analysis of computers began around 1997 with Kent Police establishing one of the first hi tech crime units in the country. More recently, the UK's National High-Tech Crime Training Centre (now part of the National Police Improvement Agency, the NPIA) has developed a number of training courses in forensic data investigation and internet investigation (at initial, intermediate and advanced levels) for investigators working both in the UK and further afield. The intention is to develop a common training model for high tech crime investigation training throughout Europe, and a linked professional register of recognised high tech crime investigators (Bryant and Jones, 2005).

3.4.1 Council for the Registration of Forensic Practitioners

The Council for the Registration of Forensic Practitioners (CRFP) was established in 1999. It is a non-profit making organisation (subsidised by a grant from the Home Office) and is independent of the Government. The Council's remit is to maintain a register of currently competent forensic practitioners and to ensure that registered practitioners stay up to date and maintain their level of competence. Initially, the register only covered the mainstream forensic specialties of science, fingerprints and scene examination, but it has been extended more recently and now includes forensic medicine, road transport investigation and fire-scene examination. Within digital forensics, the CRFP identify three processes; namely:

- Data capture;
- Data examination; and
- Data evaluation.

Data capture is the retrieval of data using forensically sound processes coupled with the creation of systems to verify the data captured. Software products such as Guidance Software's EnCase and Access Data's Forensic Toolkit (FTK) perform these two steps in one process.

The data examination role relates to the identification and examination of relevant data in an investigation. In addition, the CRFP also consider the production of exhibits (to assist the court) to be part of this role.

The data evaluation role encompasses the assessment of data in its context and assesses the significance of the data for the case in question. The forensic practitioner is also equipped to draw deductions from the data and consider alternative hypotheses.

A digital investigator may apply to join the CRFP register. The CRFP application process (at the time of writing) considers the skills of a practitioner in terms of these three roles (data capture, examination and evaluation). The application involves two separate application packs; 'Computer Examination' and 'Computers'. The data capture and examination roles fall under the Computer Examination category, as they are considered to use investigative skills. Data evaluation, which is considered to use higher level skills (similar to the skills possessed by a

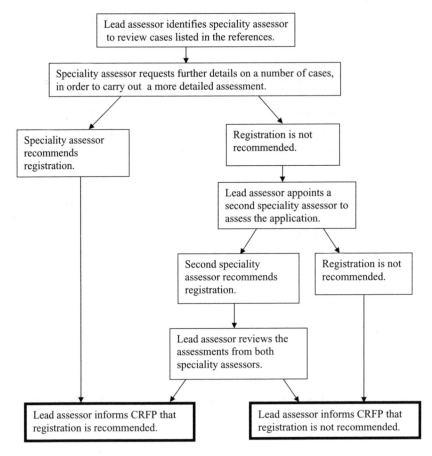

Figure 3.4 Applying for CRFP registration

forensic scientist or an engineer) is covered by the Computers application pack. A forensic examiner who undertakes all three roles (data capture, examination and evaluation) must therefore complete two application packs.

Each application is processed in three stages. In the first stage (Initial Application), the applicant returns the completed application pack(s) to the CRFP, who then obtain the relevant references for the lead assessor. The second and third stages of the application process (Further Information and Final Assessment) are shown in figure 3.4.

A successful applicant will be granted registration for 4 years. After this time has elapsed the renewal of their registration will depend upon their ability to demonstrate that they have remained up to date and maintained their competence.

In addition, the investigator's recent casework will be subjected to a further formal assessment.

Despite being based upon a system of peer review, the Seventh Report by the Select Committee on Science and Technology (Great Britain. House of Commons Science and Technology Select Committee, 2005) identified a number of potential issues with the Register. Under the present system, the discredited expert witness Professor Meadow would probably have had no difficulty in obtaining CRFP registration. Professor Meadow found himself in this situation largely due to the fact that he gave evidence in an area that was not his specialty. Solicitors and policy advisors for the CPS have also voiced concerns over the registration process as it stands, citing that there is no 'remit of evidence-based practice' and that it should not become a 'panacea for exercising a judge's discretion'.

The independent auditing of the assessment processes for granting initial accreditation and renewal of accreditation is called for, but digital forensics is a small field (compared to more established information technology based fields such as Artificial Intelligence or Software Engineering) and so the number of specialists is inevitably small. Independent auditing would consequently be difficult to arrange. As pointed out by the report, for small specialist communities like CRFP, it is inevitable that such a register will have a limited validity; members of such communities are all responsible for accrediting each other.

3.4.2 Skills for Justice

A key remit for the relevant Sector Skills Council, Skills for Justice (SfJ), is the introduction of National Occupational Standards (NOS). These standards measure an individual's competence by assessing performance in terms of nationally agreed outcomes. In terms of the investigation of digital crime, the relevant NOS are to be found within the 'Countering E-Crime' suite of competencies.

The Countering E-Crime NOS introduced by SfJ (after extensive consultation with representative employer organisations) comprises of eight units; two mandatory, one mandatory–optional and five optional.

Mandatory Units

- Identify and secure electronic evidence sources.
- Health and safety in ICT and Contact Centres.

Mandatory-Optional Units (at least one must be completed)

- Seize and record electronic evidence sources.
- Capture and preserve electronic evidence.

Optional Units (at least five must be completed)

- Seize and record electronic evidence sources.
- Capture and preserve electronic evidence.
- Investigate electronic evidence.
- Evaluate and report electronic evidence.
- Conduct internet investigations.
- Conduct network investigations.
- Working with ICT hardware and equipment.
- Technical advice and guidance.
- Security of ICT systems (Skills for Justice, 2007).

The modular, competence based approach to assessment mirrors the foundations of National Vocational Qualifications (NVQs) and Scottish Vocational Qualifications (SVQs). This approach also makes it relatively straightforward to identify areas that need further development. The distinguishing characteristics that define a successful performance (within an established role such as digital forensics) are known as competencies, reports Wolfe (1998). Any combination of knowledge, skill, traits, values/beliefs, motives, and physical ability can be assessed.

Competence based assessment is viewed by many organisations as a more suitable tool to assess workplace skills than traditional academic qualifications alone. Their modular nature makes them scaleable, meaning that as new roles are created within an organisation, appropriate competencies for the new role can be chosen from existing competencies, and additional competencies can be added to distinguish the new role from the existing role(s). Concerns however have been expressed within the academic community concerning the 'box-ticking' nature and general limitations of competencies based learning and assessment.

3.4.3 Models for professional accreditation

There is currently no professional body for digital forensic investigators and allied occupations. The establishment of a mandatory regulatory body, with the authority to issue a license to practise would help define the standards and level of expertise required of a digital forensics specialist, and courts would be likely to have greater confidence in the skills, experience and accountability of an individual specialist. It would seem rational to suppose that such a regulatory body would be led by a single voice. Without clear leadership, it is likely that prolonged debate concerning the mechanisms for arranging peer review would inevitably dilute the credibility of any professional body, defeating its very purpose.

Many professional bodies also have close ties not only with industry, but also with current research and development in order to keep abreast of the latest scientific knowledge and recommendations for best practice. The advantages for a field such as digital forensics are obvious. A regulatory body overseeing digital forensics could also cater for those with and without a higher education; the personnel working in high tech crime units within the police forces of England and Wales comprise of a mixture of both police officers and civilians with a wide range of skills and educational backgrounds.

The fingerprints service might be considered as a possible model for both professional accountability and accreditation within the forensics arena; it might provide a positive role model for other digital forensics specialities. In terms of an individual's professional accountability, fingerprints specialists are regulated by the National Fingerprint Board (NFB) which is made up of senior operational police officers, Home Office representatives and senior forensic practitioners. Standards, performance, training are all areas under the remit of the NFB.

As Mike Thompson, Head of National Fingerprint Training for Centrex (now NPIA) describes (BBC, 2006), the NFB is a regulatory body that has a mandate to enforce compliance throughout the service. A prospective fingerprint expert can expect their training to be evaluated and assessed to ensure that competence is fully proven before they can be recognised and registered as an expert. There is an ongoing process of continuous improvement and development and regular competence testing to demonstrate continuing practical competence on the part of the practitioner.

Digital Forensic Investigation

Robin Bryant

Investigating digital crime does not, of itself, mean that a digital forensic investigation will be undertaken. Some digital crimes, such as identity fraud where the suspect uses the internet as a source of information and a means to commit the crime, could feasibly be investigated entirely successfully using traditional and well established investigative techniques. However, many digital crimes also require a specialised and parallel form of digital forensic investigation. (We use the word 'forensic' here beyond its normal meaning of 'pertaining to the courts' to embrace a wider sense of scientifically-based methodologies).

The diagram below illustrates both some of the usual components of digital forensic investigation (shown in shaded boxes) although by no means all will be used in any particular investigation, together with some indication of investigative methods that span two or more subfields.

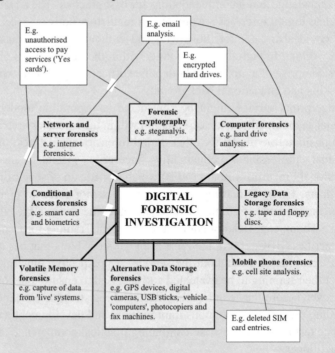

Figure 3.5 Specialist fields within digital forensic investigation

The credibility of a digital forensic analyst needs to be proven and less open to challenge, particularly given the weight that can be placed upon the digital evidence by the courts. Mechanisms need to be put in place for the review of the practices, procedures and performance for the field of study covered by a particular digital forensic analyst. In addition, the training of staff and the maintaining of standards should be demonstrable; a mandatory regulatory body could provide such mechanisms.

3.5 Digital evidence in the courts

The Office of Science and Technology states that any technical process applied to digital evidence 'does not have to pass any formal test' for it to be placed before a court (Great Britain. Parliamentary Office of Science and Technology, 2005). This may seem alarmingly imprecise, but it has certain advantages; a trial judge has the power to admit or decline a particular piece of evidence, and this flexibility allows a court to take advantage of the very latest developments in the digital forensics field.

3.5.1 Presenting digital evidence in court

The Forensic Examiner prepares a statement which is submitted to the Crown Prosecution Service (CPS), and copies are distributed to both the prosecution and defence counsel. The statement explains the examiner's findings and proposes a variety of strategies and the legal points to prove. It should not be just an unbiased and technically accurate document describing the outcome of a forensic examination; explanation and guidance should also be provided, in terms which are comprehensible to the court and witnesses.

The Forensic Examiner's primary role (as for most witnesses summoned to a court within England and Wales) is to assist the court. However, given both the technical complexity of the evidence and the examiner's level of expertise and experience, they are also frequently called upon to interpret the evidence. As Johnston and Hutton (2004) point out, the primary purpose of the statement is to assist the court in evaluating the admissibility and weight of any evidence found on the digital devices examined for the case.

Arguably the most important area to cover when presenting digital evidence to a court is that of continuity. It is absolutely critical to be able to account for what happened to an exhibit such as a computer from the moment it was seized to the moment it was examined by a forensic examiner. Any gaps in this chain of evidence could mean that one or more unknown persons could have had access to the exhibit and thus have potentially interfered with its integrity. Such discrepancies provide an easy target for defence counsel to discredit the evidence.

Under UK Law each offence has what are known as 'points to prove'. For example, under s 3 of the Computer Misuse Act 1990 a person is guilty of unauthorised modification of computer material if it can be proven that he or she:

(a) does any act which causes an unauthorised modification of the contents of any computer; and

(b) at the time when the act was performed he or she has the requisite intent and the requisite knowledge to do so.

These two points demonstrate what in legal terms is called the *actus reus* (guilty act) and the *mens rea* (intent/knowledge) of the individual.

If the evidence submitted by a digital forensics examiner is unclear or is contradicted by other evidence, the court may move to reject the examiner's evidence. R. v. Cannings (2004) (which passed judgement on Angela Canning's successful appeal against her conviction for murdering her two baby sons) it was stated that 'If the outcome of the trial depends exclusively, or almost exclusively, on a serious disagreement between distinguished and reputable experts, it will often be unwise, and therefore, unsafe to proceed' (R. v. Cannings [2004] 1 All E. R. 725).

3.5.2 Interpretation of evidence by a jury

The jury hear first the evidence of the forensic examiner as interpreted by the prosecution counsel, so it is vital that the counsel has a clear understanding of the evidence, and can communicate the key points to the jury effectively. Thus it is essential for the forensic examiner to liaise with the prosecution counsel prior to going to court, in order to check their interpretation of the facts. Such meetings, when they occur, usually take place just prior to going into court, and often only an hour at most after the prosecutor has first seen the digital forensic examiner's statement. Where appropriate, counsel is offered a carefully selected analogy to assist in the comprehension of such data.

There is a school of thought that the juries in cases involving complex digital evidence should be selected from among suitable technically qualified people. The

British Computer Society (2000) proposed this measure in a submission paper. Such a radical measure would need careful consideration as to a suitable means of establishing the degree to which a jury (under the current system) understood and appreciated the significance of evidence concerning digital devices or processes. However, conducting such research inevitably presents difficulties, as identified by section 7 of a report by the House of Commons Science and Technology Select Committee (2005) which states that 'section 8 of the Contempt of Court Act 1981 and the related common law assures the confidentiality of a jury's deliberations and precludes research into these deliberations' (Great Britain. House of Commons Science and Technology Select Committee, 2005, para 164).

3.5.3 Countering a defence

One of the responsibilities of the digital forensic examiner on the prosecution team is to identify and evaluate possible areas of defence that may arise. Probably the most common defence identified at the police interview stage of an investigation is that of a Trojan or 'pop-up' being responsible for the presence of any illegal material on the computer in question. Kennedy (2006) discusses a process that may be followed to investigate the presence and impact of malware.

In some situations a defendant may assert that evidence found on their computer was unsolicited and was 'pushed' to them via MSN, a peer-to-peer application such as Kazaa (or a BitTorrent client) or perhaps by email. These scenarios can be substantiated or refuted through investigation of the computer and how it has been used. Similar techniques can be applied to investigate claims of 'curiosity' when for example, indecent images of children are found on a computer.

The defence may argue that proper procedures have not been followed; procedure is important and must be strictly followed during a digital forensic examination. By keeping contemporaneous notes of all actions performed (particularly in relation to the technical processes followed) it is possible to demonstrate that an empirical approach has been taken to the examination of an exhibit and data contained within it. Although such notes will not find their way into a statement in their entirety they should include any areas of the ACPO guidelines that might need to be evidenced. Thus, when capturing a forensic copy of a hard disk for example, it should be recorded that the process was performed using a hardware write blocking device, and ideally record the device's manufacturer, model and serial number.

If there is a significant difference between the total number of sectors on a hard disk indicated by the label and the number of sectors reported by the analysis tool, an explanation for this difference should be provided in the statement. Without this the defence could argue that the evidence that vindicates their client is located in this 'missing' area.

3.6 Ethical issues

Digital forensics practitioners (unlike many generalist practitioners) possess the skills to access areas of a hard disk normally hidden to the other users, and this may present ethical dilemmas that can prove difficult to navigate. For example, whilst working on a high profile case a practitioner may be subject to peer pressure to release personal details of the offender to police colleagues and other investigators. The privacy of the offender or client must be maintained in exactly the same way a GP maintains the privacy of a patient, reports ComputerForensics1 (2006). For example, if a hard disk from a lawyer's office is being examined, any records of communications between the lawyer and the client are subject to what is known as 'legal privilege'. This means that such communications are regarded as confidential and must not even be examined, let alone used evidentially by a digital forensics practitioner. These privacy issues can be difficult to untangle at times as it is not always possible to confine an investigation to just one individual. For example, log files or emails between parties will by their very nature contain details such as access times and email accounts of innocent third parties.

It is not difficult to see that, like a locksmith, the digital forensic practitioner's skills can be put to misuse. In privately owned companies the use and misuse of such skills becomes more significant, reports Stahl (2006). Employers may naturally desire information about their employees, and a digital forensics practitioner may be under immense pressure to reveal particular details stored in a digital evidence source. A practitioner who submits to such pressure may stray into the realm of surveillance in the workplace; this is explored in some depth by Stahl et al. (2005).

Ethical issues should be explored alongside the provision of ethical guidance during the education and training of a practitioner, but it is not enough to simply 'bolt on' an extra subject to be covered within a digital forensics training programme. The bolt-on approach has the effect of isolating the principles, and seems to imply that it might be optional for the individual to take the concepts on board. Erbacher and Swart (2002) argue that changes in attitude such as ethics are best brought about by regularly integrating ethical considerations and discussions into all aspects of the specialty as a whole.

3.7 Professional development for digital forensics

Establishing digital forensics as a profession is an area explored by Stahl (2006), and would, Stahl asserts, provide guidance for members in the principles upheld by the profession, including ethics. As a professional body, a code of conduct can be established that embodies the expected behaviour of the profession in relation to third parties. This reduces pressure on individuals to behave in way they feel violates the principles upheld by the profession.

Stahl (2006) goes on to point out that, traditionally, members of a profession such as medicine and law are known and respected for their independence and autonomy. Employees within the newer professions such as the various flavours of information communications technology are typically employed by large commercial organisations. In these circumstances, the ethical priorities of the profession inevitably compete with the commercial priorities of the organisation. When a conflict of interest occurs it is likely the professional requirements will take second place to the commercial requirements.

The digital forensics practitioner must reflect upon the position they hold in society; they are in positions of considerable trust and power. For those working in law enforcement, there are times where the reputation and very liberty of people under investigation can depend solely upon the findings of the practitioner's examination.

Questions

Robin Bryant & Sarah Bryant

1. What is 'volatile memory'? How can the forensic 'capture' of the remains of volatile memory be reconciled with current good practice guidelines for the 'first responder'? (Compare the 'safe shutdown school' with the 'live analysis school').

2. What is a 'session cookie' and why might they be of interest to a forensic investigator?

3. In a criminal case, how could the 'trojan defence' be rebutted?

4. Describe how digital technology may contribute to the commission of a 419 scam.

5. What is the system for validating digital forensic software tools in (a) the UK, (b) the US?

6. Why might it be important to use a write blocking device in the course of a digital investigation?

7. What information is stored in a file called 'index.dat' on a PC (as used by the Microsoft web browser Internet Explorer)? Why might this information be of forensic interest?

8. What are the four principles ACPO recommends for any digital investigation?

References

Association of Chief Police Officers of England (2007) Good Practice Guide for Computer-Based Evidence. [Online]. Available at: http://www.7safe.com/electronic_evidence/ACPO_guidelines_computer_evidence.pdf (Accessed: Oct 9 2007).

BBC (2006) Q and A: The fingerprint expert. BBC News [Online]. Available at: http://news.bbc.co.uk/1/hi/programmes/panorama/5007820.stm (Accessed: Sep 9 2007).

BBC (2007a) Lawyer 'stored indecent images'. BBC News [Online]. Available at: http://news.bbc.co.uk/1/hi/england/4930898.stm (Accessed: Sep 14 2007).

BBC (2007b) Identity ring members sentenced. BBC News [Online]. Available at: http://news.bbc.co.uk/1/hi/england/london/6653727.stm (Accessed: Sep 12 2007).

BBC (2007c) Life for 'happy slap' murder boy. BBC News [Online]. Available at: http://news.bbc.co.uk/1/hi/england/southern_counties/6303599.stm (Accessed: Sep 16 2007).

BBC (2007d) Man arrested over Wi-Fi 'theft'. BBC News [Online]. Available at: http://news.bbc.co.uk/1/hi/england/london/6958429.stm (Accessed: Sep 17 2007).

BBC (2007e) Sex attack phone girls detained. BBC News [Online]. Available at: http://news.bbc.co.uk/1/hi/england/london/6970516.stm (Accessed: Sep 16 2007).

BBC (2007f) Sister jailed for identity theft. BBC News [Online]. Available at: http://news.bbc.co.uk/1/hi/scotland/edinburgh_and_east/6969221.stm (Accessed: 12 Sep 2007).

BBC (2007g) Trial hears from Special Branch. BBC News [Online]. Available at: http://news.bbc.co.uk/1/hi/scotland/tayside_and_central/6966846.stm (Accessed: Sep 6 2007).

BBC (2007h) Tutor sent to jail over ID fraud. BBC News [Online]. Available at: http://news.bbc.co.uk/1/hi/wales/south_east/6917965.stm (Accessed: 12 Sep 2007).

British Computer Society (2000) Expert Panels: Legal Affairs Expert Panel, Submission to the Criminal Courts Review, Lord Justice Auld. [Online]. Available at: http://

www.computerevidence.co.uk/Papers/LJAuld/BCSComputerEvidenceSubmission. htm (Accessed: Sep 25 2007)

Bryant, R. and Jones, N. (2005) *Cybercrime Investigation – Developing an International Training Programme for the Future.* Bedford: NSLEC Centre for National High-Tech Crime Training.

ComputerForensics1 (2006) Computer forensic ethics. [Online]. Available at: http://www.computerforensics1.com/computer-forensic-ethics.html (Accessed: Sep 10 2007).

Dhamija, R., Tygar, J.D. and Hearst, M. (2006) Why phishing works. In: Grinter, R. E., Rodden, T., Aoki, P.M., Cutrell, E., Jeffries, R. and Olson, G.M. (eds.) Proceedings of the 2006 Conference on Human Factors in Computing Systems, CHI 2006, Montréal, Québec, Canada: CHI, pp. 581–590.

Erbacher, R.F. and Swart, R.S. (2002) *Computer forensics: training and education.* [Online]. Available at: http://www.cs.usu.edu/~erbacher/publications/ForensicsEducationPaperrevised.pdf (Accessed: Sep 10 2007).

Garlik Limited (2007) UK Cybercrime report. [Online]. Available at: https://www.garlik.com/press/Garlik_UK_Cybercrime_Report.pdf (Accessed: Sep 11 2007).

Great Britain. House of Commons Science and Technology Select Committee (2005) Science and Technology – Seventh Report: (Chapter 7 Use of Forensic Evidence in Court), London: HMSO. [Online]. Available at: http://www.publications.parliament.uk/pa/cm200405/cmselect/cmsctech/96/9610.htm (Accessed: Sep 9 2007).

Great Britain. Office of Public Sector Information (2006) Explanatory Notes to Fraud Act 2006. London: HMSO. [Online]. Available at: http://www.opsi.gov.uk/ACTS/en2006/2006en35.htm (Accessed: 03 Sep 2007).

Great Britain. Parliamentary Office of Science and Technology (2005) Postnote – Science in Court. [Online]. Available at: http://www.parliament.uk/documents/upload/postpn248.pdf#search=%22presenting%20digital%20evidence%20court%22 (Accessed: 26 Sep 2006).

Guardian news and Media Limited (2005) Concern over rise of 'happy slapping' craze. [Online]. Available at: http://www.guardian.co.uk/mobile/article/0,2763,1470214,00.html (Accessed: Sep 16 2007).

Guardian news and Media Limited (2007) Love in the time of phone porn. [Online]. Available at: http://education.guardian.co.uk/sexeducation/story/0,,2001374,00.html (Accessed: Sep 14 2007).

International Centre for Nigerian Law (2007) Criminal code act part VI. [Online]. Available at: http://www.nigeria-law.org/Criminal%20Code%20Act-Part%20VI%20%20to%20the%20end.htm (Accessed: 3 Sep 2007).

Johnston, D. and Hutton, G. (2004) *Blackstone's Police Manual, Evidence and Procedure.* Oxford: Oxford University Press, p. 133.

Kennedy, I.M. (2006) It was a big wooden horse, your Honour. [Online]. Available at: http://www.bcs.org/server.php?show=ConWebDoc.6232 (Accessed: Sep 27 2006).

O'Connell, R. (2007) A typology of child cybersexploitation and online grooming practices. Lancashire: University of Central Lancashire, 24 July 2003, [Online]. Available at: http://www.uclan.ac.uk/host/cru/docs/cru010.pdf (Accessed: Sep 24 2007).

Skills for Justice (2007) National Occupational Standards for the Justice Sector. [Online]. Available at: http://www.skillsforjustice.com/nos/with-ple.htm (Accessed 10 Oct 2007).

Stahl, B.C. (2006) Is forensic computing a profession? Revisiting an old debate in a new field. *Journal of Digital Forensics, Security and Law,* **1**(4):49–66 [Online]. Available at: http://www.cse.dmu.ac.uk/~bstahl/publications/2006_forensic_computing_profession_JDFSL.pdf (Accessed: Sep 10 2007).

Stahl, B.C., Prior, M., Wilford, S. and Dervla, C. (2005) Electronic monitoring in the workplace: if people don't care, then what is the relevance? In: Weckert, J. (ed.) *Electronic Monitoring in the Workplace: Controversies and Solutions*. USA: Idea-Group Publishing, pp. 50–78.

Symantec Corporation (2007a) A Monster Trojan. [Online]. Available at: http://www.symantec.com/enterprise/security_response/weblog/2007/08/a_monster_trojan.html (Accessed: Sep 12 2007).

Symantec Corporation (2007b) Symantec Internet Security Threat Report. [Online]. Available at:http://eval.symantec.com/mktginfo/enterprise/white_papers/ent-white-paper_internet_security_threat_report_xii_09_2007.en-us.pdf (Accessed: Sep 17 2007).

Thornton, J. (1997) The general assumptions and rationale of forensic identification. In: Faigman, D.L., Kaye, D.H., Saks, M.J. and Sanders, J. (eds.) *Modern Scientific Evidence: The Law And Science Of Expert Testimony* **2**. St. Paul: West Publishing Co.

Wolfe, M. (1998) Transitioning to a competency for pay system. *Conference Proceedings of Linkage Incorporated, USA* **5**:203–279.

4

Countering Cybercrime

Denis Edgar-Nevill and Paul Stephens

In this chapter we examine the response to cybercrime at the level of both government and law enforcement agencies and at the level of the individual consumer
or PC user.

4.1 Recognising digital crime as something new

In 1951 J. Lyons & Co., the UK's leading bakery and catering firm began operating
the 'Lyons Electronic Office' computer, capable of around 700 instructions a
second with a massive (for the time) 4 kb of main memory. This was the first
commercial business use of a computer anywhere in the World (Bird, 1994).
Ever since, criminal minds have sought new ways of unlawfully manipulating
computers and their software systems.

But is it something new? Isn't it just crime? Do we need to do anything more
than just prosecute offenders using existing laws and good, old-fashioned police
work? Clearly creating new legislation is time-consuming and expensive; it makes
an already complicated situation more complex (why put 'old wine in new bottles'? (Grabosky, 2001)) and is unnecessary, if an existing law will suit.

In the 1970s the ability to remotely access computers using just a home computer and a modem saw the first instances of 'hacking'. For the price of a telephone call (or nothing if the hacker accessed the telephone company's computer

Investigating Digital Crime   Edited by Robin Bryant and Sarah Bryant
© 2008 John Wiley & Sons, Ltd

and cancelled the bill) hackers potentially had access to machines all around the world. As mentioned elsewhere in this book, one of the first people convicted of a hacking offence was the infamous 'Captain Crunch' who discovered a means to duplicate the tones used on AT&T phone lines. He used a breakfast cereal toy in Cap'n Crunch Cereal (hence the sobriquet) to produce a tone of 2600 Hz which mimicked the AT&T trunk-line disconnection process. He produced a blue box mimicking a range of other telephone signals (see Chapter 8 for further details) and was prosecuted and sentenced in October 1972 to 5 years' probation for toll fraud (World News, 2007).

There was no specific need for the introduction of new legislation for this particular type of crime. But other types of hack are perhaps different in nature; new and different forms of crime (possibly 'new wine in no bottles'? (Wall, 1999)).

'Loveball' cyberfraud

Robin Bryant

An example of a digital crime which is clearly also a cybercrime (and perhaps could be termed a 'cyberfraud') occurred in Portugal in November 2000. Portuguese police were alerted to complaints from individuals who had run up large telephone bills for a premium rate telephone service that he or she had never intentionally used. The itemised charges on the telephone bills related to 'Audiotext' messages charged at 659 escudos (approximately €3.25) per minute. By the end of the enquiry Portuguese police had received over 4 000 complaints.

After initial investigations, the police established that all the complainants had also accessed one (or both) of two internet sites specialising in adult pornography. The complainants had been made aware of the existence of these sites through advertisements, such as 'pop-ups' (appearing whilst using an internet browser), and had accessed the internet sites in the normal way, that is through his or her ISP (at 12 escudos per minute). It was therefore unclear what connection there was (if any) between the two internet websites and a premium rate telephone line.

Further investigation revealed that when a viewer agreed to enter either of the websites he or she was prompted to download a small program that would allow the pornographic images on offer to be viewed. This program was in reality a dial-up program which installed itself on the user's PC and placed a shortcut icon on the Windows desktop. Double-clicking on this icon would seamlessly but secretly perform the following actions:

1. Turn the modem sound off (if it was set to 'on');

2. Disconnect the user from the internet;

3. Reconnect the user to a different ISP carrying the website, but now through a premium rate telephone number;

4. Allow access to the material offered.

When the user finally navigated away from the sites, the above procedure would be reversed (again without the user's knowledge), reconnecting to the previous (and non premium rate) ISP. However, the user was charged whilst accessing the pornographic websites at the equivalent of €190 per hour, and most of this was received by the individuals running the scam.

Portuguese police used the program 'Winhex' to examine the code used in the secret dial-up program, and finally established (using 'Whois' tools) the identity and location of the fraudsters involved. A total of four people (Dutch, Mexican, Slovenian and Portuguese) from a company employing 20 people were arrested and prosecuted. It was estimated that the fraud yielded approximately €4 million for those involved before arrests were made.

Sources:

Expresso (2002) *PJ desmonta fraude de milhões na Net*.[Online]. Available at: http://members.fortunecity.com/botabaxo/pais411.html. (Accessed: Oct 20 2007).

Ó Ciardhuáin, S. & Gillen, P. (2002) *Training: Cyber Crime Investigation – Guide to Best Practice*. Project No. JAI/2001/Falcone/127. Dublin: An Garda Síochána.

4.2 The inadequacy of existing law

Around 18.00 local time on 3 November 1988 Robert T. Morris, a graduate student at Cornell University, released the first computer 'worm' (a form of computer virus that aggressively invades computer systems by breaking passwords and exploiting security flaws in operating systems). The worm spread rapidly through the internet infecting thousands of computers and compromising and degrading the global performance of the internet. The repair bill for each machine infected, amounted to between $200 and in excess of $53 000. He was put on probation for three years and sentenced to 400 hours of community service and a $10 050 fine, with a further $3 275 to cover the cost of his probation supervision. Clearly, the fine did not match the multi-million dollar clean-up bill; the sentence was considered by many to be incommensurate with the damage caused and not much of a deterrent to others who might follow.

As Tracey Stevens noted in Chapter 2, in the mid 1980s Robert Schifreen and Stephen Gold were alleged to have gained unauthorised access to British Telecom's Prestel interactive Viewdata service and the private personal message box of the Duke of Edinburgh, using a home computer and a modem. The defendants were arrested and charged with defrauding BT by manufacturing a 'false instrument', referring to the internal condition of BT's equipment after it had processed Gold's eavesdropped password. Tried in the Southwark Crown Court under s 1 of the Forgery and Counterfeiting Act 1981, they were convicted (R. v. Gold and Schifreen, HL 21 April 1988) on specimen charges (five against Schifreen, four against Gold) and fined. Although the fines were only small, the defendants decided to appeal to the Criminal Division of the Court of Appeal, citing the lack of evidence proving that they had attempted to obtain material gain from their actions, and claiming that the Counterfeiting Act had been misapplied in their case ([1988] AC 1063). They were acquitted by the Lord Justice Lane. The prosecution appealed to the House of Lords in 1988 which affirmed the acquittal.

In essence the only tangible thing stolen by Schifreen and Gold might have been said to be the minuscule amounts of electricity involved in the password and data transfers, so no real mechanism to prosecute them was available to law enforcement agencies. At the time this decision was greeted as a 'Hackers' Charter' in the UK.

Cybercrime moved into the realm of billion dollar damages in May 2000 when the 'Love Bug' infected over 270 000 computers worldwide in the first few hours after its release. It was sent by email with a message header 'I Love You', and when the email was opened it destroyed certain types of files on the computer and emailed itself onto other users using the addresses in the computer's mailbox. The message header proved so enticing to many recipients that the effect of the virus included shutting down large companies such as the Ford Motor Company in the USA, and notably the House of Lords in the UK. The Love Bug is estimated to have caused $10 billion of damage (disinfection of machines and productivity lost) in 20 countries. In the Philippines, where no specific computer crime legislation existed at the time, an attempt was made to prosecute the offenders under credit card law but this was dropped.

The Love Bug illustrates the new problems that cybercrime brings:

- The lack of cybercrime-specific laws and/or the inadequacy of existing legislation; laws that were crafted to deal with criminal conduct occurring in the real, physical world, not in or by means of the virtual world of cyberspace;

- The lack of international agreements on cybercrime;

- The difficulty of ascertaining which nation(s) has/have jurisdiction to prosecute a cyber-criminal and, once this determination has been made, of asserting jurisdiction over that person;

- The difficulty of determining how many offences have been committed, against whom and the damage resulting from those offences (Brenner, 2001).

Gradually, as the damage and inconvenience from cybercrime spreads to affect potentially everyone in the community, the public image of the computer hacker/software virus creator has changed from that of a super-intelligent, fun person, to that of a nuisance or potential criminal.

4.3 What is cybercrime?

If we are dealing with something new (which current evidence suggests is true) then exactly what is it? We know it has developed and taken shape on the margins, and that it overlaps a range of different disciplines (Figure 4.1).

Agreeing a definition of cybercrime is more problematic. Some definitions simply focus on the financial aspects of cybercrime; for example, 'Crimes perpetrated over the internet, typically having to do with online fraud' (Techweb, 2007), or 'Cybercrime is the use of computers and the internet by criminals to perpetrate fraud and other crimes against companies and consumers' (Z2Z, 2007).

Clearly cybercrime (or 'cyber crime') is more than this. Some definitions which try to elaborate develop instead into lists; for example:

> Cyber crime encompasses any criminal act dealing with computers and networks (called hacking). Additionally, cyber crime also includes traditional crimes conducted through the Internet. For example; hate

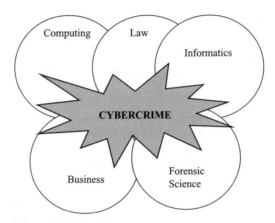

Figure 4.1 Cybercrime emerges as a new discipline (Edgar-Nevill, 2007a)

crimes, telemarketing and Internet fraud, identity theft, and credit card account thefts are considered to be cyber crimes when the illegal activities are committed through the use of a computer and the Internet. Webopedia.Com (Webopedia, 2007)

It is doubtful whether such definitions are particularly helpful as the forms of cybercrime vary and change with every new way that computer technology is exploited. Definitions of cybercrime quite often settle for a compromise between listing certain crimes and general statements; for example, 'Noun 1. cybercrime – crime committed using a computer and the internet to steal a person's identity or sell contraband or stalk victims or disrupt operations with malevolent programs' (Princeton University, 2007) and thefreedictionary (TFD, 2007).

Perhaps Wall is right when he suggests that the term 'cybercrime' tends to be used '... metaphorically and emotionally rather than scientifically or legally...' and is fairly meaningless (Wall, 2007, p. 10). Do we really need to agree on a definition to enact legislation? Clearly the answer is 'no'. For example, the first legislation to address computer crime in the UK (the Computer Misuse Act 1990) uses the term 'computer' many times but at no point defines what the term 'computer' means. However, being imprecise about the exact meaning of terms used could present problems for courts, regarding the interpretation of legislation. For example, does the term 'computer' include the *Oxford English Dictionary* definition which includes references to people whose task is to calculate (OED, 2007)? This is a pre-electronic definition of the term, which would clearly not be considered as relevant within the context of modern computer law.

4.4 Legislation and law enforcement

The proposed changes and additions to the Computer Misuse Act 1990 (CMA), largely as a result of the Police and Justice Act 2006, are discussed in Chapter 2. The new offences created under the CMA will extend the law and criminalise those who make, supply or receive software or hardware tools to commit offences (BBC, 2007d). However, the wording of the Act is so general that some experts in the field, such as Adam Laurie, are concerned that this could compromise anyone endeavouring to identify the flaws in computer systems, including those people who act with the sole intention of improving security for everyone, and with no malicious intent (Laurie, 2007). Only time, and accumulating case law, will tell if his fears are justified.

Some countries have been a little slower than the UK and others in passing legislation to cover cybercrime (for example Sri Lanka published its legislation in July 2007; Computer Crime Act July 2007 (Zoysa *et al.*, 2007)).

4.4.1 Police training and digital crime

There is some evidence that governments and law enforcement agencies have been ill-prepared to meet the challenges of cybercrime, even when the legislation exists. The European Information Society Group (EURIM) published a third discussion paper in 2004 as part of the IPPR E-Crime Study drafted by UK MPs, entitled 'Supplying the Skills for Justice: addressing the needs of law enforcement and industry for investigatory and enforcement skills'. In this discussion paper the following point is made:

> We have around 140 000 police officers in the UK. Barely 1000 have been trained to handle digital evidence at the basic level and fewer than 250 of them are currently with Computer Crime Units or have higher-level forensic skills. (EURIM, 2004)

There has certainly been a growth in training programmes developed by national police training agencies, for example the National Policing Improvement Agency (NPIA, 2007) in the UK, and a parallel growth in the numbers of universities offering undergraduate and postgraduate programmes; Canterbury Christ Church University (CCCU, 2005), Cranfield University (Cranfield, 2007), University of Glamorgan (Glamorgan, 2007), Northumbria University (Northumbria, 2007) to name but a few. However, because of the comparatively small numbers of people with appropriate expertise, the number of offences far outweighs the available investigative resources, and severely restricts the number of successful prosecutions.

SOCA

The most important national development in the UK has been the establishment of the SOCA (Serious Organised Crime Agency) in 2006 (SOCA, 2007). Dubbed 'Britain's FBI' by Tony Blair (BBC, 2006a), the agency is an amalgam of the National Crime Squad, the National Criminal Intelligence Service (NCIS), and investigators from Customs and the Home Office's Immigration Service (UKIS). It is an executive non-departmental public body sponsored by, but operationally independent from, the Home Office. Its important strategic priorities identified by the Government were:

- SOCA should devote a higher proportion of its resources and activity to intelligence work than the agencies that it replaces;

- Class A drugs and organised immigration crime, in that order, should be its top priorities;

- effort should continue to be devoted also to the other organised crime threats already identified, including fraud against individuals and the private sector, high tech crime, counterfeiting, the use of firearms and serious robbery; and

- emphasis should be placed on recovering the proceeds of crime.

(SOCA, 2007)

Superficially, there are clear advantages to establishing such a high-level organisation, as it should simplify the process of international liaison and coordination in order to fight serious crime. Indeed, SOCA has already been instrumental in the breaking of international drugs operations (BBC, 2006b, 2007b, 2007c). However, there have been some suggestions that gaps are appearing in the UK's ability to fight cybercrime (Espiner, 2007). As part of its formation SOCA replaced the National Hi-Tech Crime Unit (NHTCU). Now it seems that a gap may be developing between the skills required to tackle highest level crime considered by SOCA and the capabilities, capacities and expertise available to regional police forces in the UK (The Register, 2007).

4.5 Challenges

The main public focus on cybercrime still relates to paedophilia and offences against children. However, cybercrime is not just sexual crime facilitated by the internet but a whole spectrum of activities, including copyright infringement, harassment, blackmail, identity theft, denial of services, theft of data, and large and small-scale fraud. The British Crime Survey does not include statistical information specifically referring to computer related crime in its main body but does refer to criminal activity facilitated by computers, such as fraud, in associated reports (BBC, 2007a). Financial organisations are reluctant to publish statistics in this area, as are many victims of such crimes, possibly because the sums are small and there is a delay between deciding to purchase online and the expected receipt of goods, maybe weeks later. The apparent number of offences is also reduced due to the difficulties encountered by police forces when pursuing investigations involving perpetrators in other counties covered by other police forces. These factors would apply particularly for offences that individually involve small sums of money (Bracey and Edgar-Nevill, 2007).

Detective Chief Inspector Charlie McMurdie of the London's Metropolitan Police specialist crime directorate was the author of a report (McMurdie, 2007) which considered:

- the need for a new national police body to tackle e-crime (despite the existence of SOCA);

- the difficulties faced by individual UK police forces in keeping pace with the volumes of crime; to the point where e-crimes are not investigated 'due to the volume of offences and the national and international nature of e-crime, sometimes involving hundreds or thousands of victims ...';

- the low prosecution rate of hackers; police are trying to keep pace with hackers who have evolved from enthusiastic amateur criminals into '... financially motivated, organized global criminal enterprises.'

The majority of the 43 police forces in the UK have a high tech crime unit (sometimes as part of a larger investigation unit or group, sometimes with a different name) but these units frequently have a significant backlog of cases (up to a year) and they inevitably concentrate on very serious offences such as child pornography and paedophilia which typically require up to 80 per cent of their time. As computer systems become larger and more complex, and criminals more experienced (and expert) in employing more sophisticated techniques, law enforcement presents an ever increasing challenge.

We should also be mindful that the responsibility for addressing cybercrime is a collective one; not something that can (or should) be left to any one agency. This was the subject of a House of Lords Science and Technology Committee report that observed that a type of 'Wild West' culture prevails in relation to the internet, and that users are left to protect themselves. Lord Broers (2007), chairman of the House of Lords Science and Technology Committee concluded that:

> You can't just rely on individuals to take responsibility for their own security. They will always be out-foxed by the bad guys. We feel many of the organisations profiting from internet services now need to take their share of the responsibility. That includes the IT industry and the software vendors, the banks and internet traders, and ISPs.

4.6 Individual responsibilities

There are a number of ways in which the vulnerability of small computer systems to cybercrime may be reduced. The smaller systems, typically found in homes and small offices are likely to have been set up and run by people without any professional IT training, and these systems are particularly vulnerable to criminal exploitation by unauthorised users.

All users want a computer system that is easy to use but secure to outside threats. Unfortunately, there is usually a conflict between ease of use and security. The more secure a computer system is, the harder it is to use and vice versa. Operating systems for home users have historically focused on ease of use, and although this is changing, third party software is still required before a computer system can be considered safe for online use. Software companies and Internet Service Providers (ISPs) proclaim the excellence of new security features, but frequently supply internet connection equipment with only the minimum of security features enabled. Users are generally unaware that such security features must be enabled in order to provide security; users quite often wrongly assume that a computer is just like any other household appliance and that connecting a computer system to the internet is just like plugging in any other kind of electrical equipment. This is not the case, and in order to remain secure when using a computer on the internet some ease of use must be sacrificed.

The reason for this sacrifice is that malicious programs and deliberate attackers are constantly scanning computers connected to the internet for vulnerabilities.

Attackers may want to (amongst other reasons):

- store illicit or illegal files on a user's hard disk;
- attack another computer system through a user's internet connection; or
- steal a user's personal details, to perpetrate identity theft and fraud.

When dial-up modems were the norm, this risk of attack was reduced as connections were relatively slow and of short duration; few people were connected to the internet for any great length of time. Asymmetric Digital Subscriber line (ADSL), more commonly known as broadband, has changed this and users now have fast connections, and are permanently connected online.

4.6.1 User account permissions

Surfing the internet when logged on to the system using the administrator account is potentially a major security flaw. This is because the 'administrator' has a high level of control over the computer in use, including the ability to install new programs, change file permissions and passwords, and delete any files. If the user inadvertently installs a piece of malicious software ('malware') by clicking on a hyperlink, the unwanted software will be run with all the administrator privileges.

To avoid such problems, an account with restricted permissions should be created for each user. If a piece of malware is encountered, a user account will probably not have sufficient rights to install or run it properly. The disadvantage of an account with restricted permissions is that on occasions, it will not run a program, and the user will need to switch to a different user account.

4.6.2 Passwords

Most operating systems and websites require a user to log on using a username and password. Many people make the following mistakes when choosing and using their passwords:

- default passwords are left unchanged;
- passwords chosen are too short; and
- dictionary words are chosen.

Password-cracking tools are available to automatically try a wide range of combinations. All computer users should bear in mind that usernames, spouse's name, children's names, phone numbers and vehicle registration numbers are all pieces of information that are easily available to an attacker.

It is normally advised that passwords should include at least seven characters, using upper and lower case letters, and at least one special character, such as an asterisk. The same password should not be used for all computers and websites; otherwise if one is compromised, all will be. However, a user must be able to remember a password and not resort to the alternative strategy of jotting down passwords on sticky notes to adorn the monitor! Microsoft (2007a) for example, offers some sensible suggestions for choosing a strong password and rates how strong or weak a password is (Microsoft, 2007b with an inevitable disclaimer). Chapter 5 considers passwords in more detail.

4.6.3 Software vulnerabilities

Operating systems and software applications will occasionally contain a vulnerability that could potentially be used by an attacker to gain some or total control of a computer. Even the most inexperienced attacker (also known as a 'script kiddie') can exploit these vulnerabilities if they remain unfixed.

Fortunately, most software manufacturers regularly release system and application updates, known as 'patches'. Microsoft Windows^{TM} offers an automatic updates facility to automatically install and run such patches. Alternatively, a user may prefer to visit Microsoft's (2007c) update site and perform the relevant updates manually.

4.6.4 Spyware

Spyware is a piece of software that is usually installed without the user's knowledge. It allows someone other than the user of the computer to remotely monitor the user's activity. This can include listing websites visited, and for how long a user views a particular site. Such information is then generally used for advertising and marketing purposes; this particular type of spyware is referred to as 'adware'. In its most innocuous form, spyware takes the form of a 'tracking cookie', recording user preferences based on the user's browsing history. For example, if a user visits a website about football, he or she may find that adverts on websites visited subsequently are tailored to advertise football-related goods. Companies may share cookies in order to target individual users with tailored advertising.

More sinister forms of spyware involve programs that run in the background without the user's knowledge. Some users may give their 'permission' in a very general sense of 'allowing cookies', without fully appreciating the implications of their decision. This sort of spyware tends to be packaged with other software installed by a user, such as peer-to-peer filesharing software or free games. Sometimes the user agrees to install spyware (though it is not termed as such) as part of the license agreement for newly acquired software. However, it is likely that many people will not be inclined to read long and complex license documents and many sites do not even require the reader to scroll to the end before providing an 'I agree' click box.

In addition to the invasion of privacy, this kind of software may have other consequences for the computer user; spyware can cause a computer system to run more slowly or even to crash. This is because it is using the computer's memory and network connection to send data to the software originator, reducing the processing power and memory capacity of the afflicted computer.

Many software manufacturers now produce anti-spyware products and indeed many come bundled with anti-virus packages. Some of the more popular and free stand-alone solutions include Grisoft AVG Anti-Spyware Free (Grisoft AVG, 2007), Lavasoft Ad-Aware SE Personal (Lavasoft, 2007), and Spybot Search & Destroy (Spybot, 2007). Another way to protect against the proliferation of spyware is to switch from a standard browser (such as Microsoft's Internet Explorer) to one that purports to offer greater security such as Mozilla Firefox (Mozilla, 2007a). The company claims that 'Firefox will not allow a Web site to download, install, or run programs on your computer without your explicit agreement. Period' (Mozilla, 2007b).

4.6.5 Malware

Malware is any piece of software devised with malicious intent. Spyware is one form of malware; however there are other kinds of malicious software such as 'Trojans', 'viruses' and 'worms'. Blended attacks (such as CodeRed and Bugbear) use several different types of malware in combination.

A 'Trojan' or 'Trojan horse', is named after the infamous gift to the city of Troy. Ancient Greek mythology recounts that a wooden horse left by the Greeks (ostensibly as a gift) was hollow, and full of experienced warriors ready to launch an attack; a computer Trojan contains a similarly unpleasant surprise. In simple terms, a Trojan is an apparently useful program that conceals a hidden function; a picture viewer application could also contain monitoring software. The software installs itself and subsequently logs every keystroke made, and transmits this information to the originator of the software.

A 'virus' is a computer program that attaches itself to legitimate files, though the term is frequently used to identify all forms of malware. Viruses tend to cause disruptive or unexpected events such as the deletion of all photographic files. They are spread by email or over a network, often by sending the infected file. A 'worm' is often confused with a virus. A worm is self-replicating but differs from a virus in that it does need to use a file to travel from system to system.

Many anti-virus products (such as Sophos (2007) and F-Secure (2007)) are readily available on the market. Companies may also offer free versions, but users should be aware that some features in the free version may be disabled and updates may not be as extensive or frequent. The anti-virus product should be updated by the user frequently, at least once a day. Alternatively, the software can be set to update automatically. It is also advisable to scan the hard drive on a regular basis, at least weekly, and periodically identify and review the processes running. Internet search engines such as Google are useful tools for helping to identify any malware that may have been inadvertently installed.

4.6.6 Firewalls

A computer with no firewall (or a badly configured firewall) is effectively advertising the programs that are running and hence available to a potential attacker. Windows XP^{TM} is supplied with its own firewall but there are also other software firewalls, such as ZoneAlarm (2007) which act as a filter between a PC and the outside world. When properly configured, ZoneAlarm prevents access to a computer by unauthorised users and applications, and prohibits others from knowing which programs are running. It allows a user to select the programs which are to have access to the internet and to select which users and applications should have access to the user's PC.

However, users may struggle to understand some of the alerts provided by a personal software firewall, and a poorly configured firewall may interfere or even block certain applications.

Questions

Robin Bryant & Sarah Bryant

1. What steps could carers take to increase the security of their children whilst online?

2. How far is security in cyberspace the joint responsibility of government, ISPs, law enforcement agencies and the individual?

3. What organisation incorporated (inter alia) the National Crime Squad, the National Criminal Intelligence Service (NCIS), and investigators from Customs and the Home Office's Immigration Service?

4. What risks are associated with accessing the internet through the administrator account on a PC?

5. Why is selecting a word from the dictionary a risky strategy for choosing a password?

6. For what reasons do some companies use spyware?

7. What are two reasons why a home PC user might not use a firewall on his or her PC?

References

BBC (2006a) Agency 'to target brutal crime'. BBC News [Online]. Available at: http://news.bbc.co.uk/1/hi/uk/4870988.stm (Accessed: Sep 26 2007).

BBC (2006b) Plymouth ship in £60m drugs bust. BBC News [Online]. Available at: http://news.bbc.co.uk/1/hi/england/devon/6126032.stm (Accessed: Sep 26 2007).

BBC (2007a) Government 'must act on e-crime'. BBC News [Online]. Available at: http://news.bbc.co.uk/1/hi/technology/6938796.stm (Accessed: Sep 26 2007).

BBC (2007b) Couple 'at centre' of drugs ring. BBC News [Online]. Available at: http://news.bbc.co.uk/1/hi/scotland/tayside_and_central/6317333.stm (Accessed: Sep 26 2007).

BBC (2007c) Drug smuggler ordered to pay £1m. BBC News [Online]. Available at: http://news.bbc.co.uk/1/hi/england/bristol/6994650.stm (Accessed: Sep 26 2007).

BBC (2007d) Cyber crime tool kits go on sale. BBC News [Online]. Available at: http://news.bbc.co.uk/1/hi/technology/6976308.stm (Accessed: Sep 26 2007).

Bird, P.J. (1994) *LEO: The First Business Computer*. Wokingham: Hasler Publishing Co.

Bracey, C. and Edgar-Nevill, D. (2007) Prosecuting Low-level Cybercrime in the UK. Proceedings of the 1st International Conference on Cybercrime Forensics Education and Training CFET 2007, Canterbury Christ Church University.

Brenner, S. (2001) Cybercrime Investigation and Prosecution: The Role of Penal and Procedural Law. *Murdoch University Electronic Journal of Law* [Online]. Available at: http://www.murdoch.edu.au/elaw/issues/v8n2/brenner82.html (Accessed: Sep 26 2007).

Broers, Lord (2007) Government must act now to maintain confidence in the internet – Lords Science and Technology Committee. [Online]. Available at: http://www.parliament.uk/parliamentary_committees/lords_press_notices/pn100807st.cfm (Accessed: Oct 10 2007).

CCCU (2005) Canterbury Christ Church joins forces with central police training and development authority to deliver masters degree in cybercrime forensics. [Online]. Available at: http://www.canterbury.ac.uk/news/newsRelease.asp?newsPk=517 (Accessed: Jun 15 2007)

Cranfield (2007) Forensic Computing MSc/PgDip/PgCert. [Online]. Available at: http://www.dcmt.cranfield.ac.uk/prospectus/postgraduate/computing (Accessed: Sep 26 2007).

Edgar-Nevill, D. (2007a) Work-Based Blended Learning through University Partnerships: A Case Study in Cybercrime Forensics. IERA2007 International Employment Relations Association 15th Annual Conference, Canterbury Christ Church University Jul 8–13 2007.

Edgar-Nevill, D. (2007b) Motivating & Engaging Forensic Computing Practitioners in Higher Education. *Innovations in Lifelong Learning Conference*, Birkbeck Institute for Lifelong Learning, Birkbeck, University of London, Jun 29 2007.

Espiner, T. (2007) Police: We're overwhelmed by e-crime. [Online]. Available at: http://news.zdnet.co.uk/security/0,1000000189,39285631,00.htm (Accessed: Sep 26 2007).

EURIM (2004) EURIM–IPPR E-Crime Study Partnership Policing for the Information Society Third Discussion Paper Supplying the Skills for Justice : Addressing the needs of law enforcement and industry. [Online]. Available at: http://www.eurim.org/consult/e-crime/may_04/ECS_DP3_Skills_040505_web.htm (Accessed: Sep 26 2007).

F-Secure (2007) F-Secure.com > F-Secure Corporation protects consumers and businesses against computer viruses and other threats. [Online]. Available at: http://www.f-secure.com/ (Accessed: July 11 2007).

Glamorgan School of Computing (2007) [Online]. Available at: http://www.glam.ac.uk/soc/ (Accessed: Sep 26 2007).

Grabosky, P. (2001) Virtual criminality, old wine in new bottles. *Social and Legal Studies* 10(2):243–249.

Grisoft AVG (2007) AVG Free Advisor – AVG Anti-Spyware Free Edition. [Online]. Available at: :http://free.grisoft.com/doc/20/us/frt/0 (Accessed: July 11 2007).

Laurie (2007) RFIDIOts!!!– Practical RFID hacking (without soldering irons or patent attorneys). Proceedings of the 1st International Conference on Cybercrime Forensics Education and Training CFET 2007, Canterbury Christ Church University.

Lavasoft (2007) Ad-aware 2007 Free – Lavasoft. [Online]. Available at: http://www. lavasoftusa.com/products/ad_aware_free.php (Accessed: July 11 2007).

McMurdie, C. (2007) Progress of MPS e-crime strategy. Metropolitan Police Service [Online]. Available at: http://www.mpa.gov.uk/committees/mpa/2007/070125/10.htm (Accessed: Sep 26 2007).

Microsoft Corporation (2007a) Strong passwords: How to create and use them. [Online]. Available at: http://www.microsoft.com/protect/yourself/password/create.mspx (Accessed: Jul 11 2007).

Microsoft Corporation (2007b) Password checker. [Online]. Available at: http://www. microsoft.com/protect/yourself/password/checker.mspx (Accessed: Jul 11 2007).

Microsoft Corporation (2007c) Microsoft Windows Update. [Online]. Available at: http://www.update.microsoft.com/microsoftupdate/v6/default.aspx?ln=en-us (Accessed: Jul 11 2007).

Mozilla (2007a) Mozilla Firefox in English – Mozilla Europe. [Online]. Available at: http://www.mozilla-europe.org/en/products/firefox/ (Accessed: Jul 11 2007).

Mozilla (2007b) Mozilla Firefox – Main Features – Mozilla Europe. [Online]. Available at: http://www.mozilla-europe.org/en/products/firefox/features/#secure (Accessed: Jul 11 2007).

Northumbria University (2007) Unique collaboration in computer forensics. [Online]. Available at: http://northumbria.ac.uk/browse/ne/uninews/564007 (Accessed: Sep 26 2007).

NPIA (2007) National Policing Improvement Agency. [Online]. Available at: http://www.npia.police.uk/ (Accessed: Sep 26 2007).

OED (2007) *Oxford English Dictionary.* [Online]. Available at: http://dictionary.oed. com/cgi/lclogin (Accessed: Sep 26 2007).

Princeton University (2007) WordNet Search. [Online]. Available at: http://wordnet. princeton.edu/perl/webwn?s=Cybercrime&o2=&o0=1&o7=&o5=&o1=1&o6=&o4= &o3=&h= (Accessed: Sep 26 2007).

SOCA (2007) Serious Organised Crimes Agency. [Online]. Available at: http://www.soca.gov.uk/aboutUs/index.html (Accessed: Sep 26 2007).

Sophos (2007) Sophos – anti-virus and anti-spam software for businesses. [Online]. Available at: http://www.sophos.com/ (Accessed: Jul 11 2007).

Spybot (2007) Downloads – The home of Spybot S&D. [Online]. Available at: http:// www.safer-networking.org/en/download/ (Accessed: Jul 11 2007).

Techweb (2007) TechEncyclopedia. Techweb.com. [Online]. Available at: http:// www.techweb.com/encyclopedia/defineterm.jhtml?term=cybercrime&x=0&y=0 (Accessed: Sep 26 2007).

TFD (2007) TheFreeDictionary. [Online]. Available at: http://www.thefreedictionary. com/cybercrime (Accessed: Sep 26 2007).

The Register (2007) London police can't cope with cybercrime. The Register 1st February 2007 [Online]. Available at: http://www.theregister.co.uk/ 2007/02/01/london_police_cybercrime/ (Accessed: Sep 26 2007).

Wall, D.S. (1999) Cybercrimes: new wine, no bottles? In: Davies, P., Francis, P. and Jupp, V. (eds) *Invisible Crimes: Their Victims and Their Regulation.* Basingstoke: Macmillan.

Wall, D.S. (2007) *Cybercrime.* Cambridge: Polity.

Webopedia (2007) Webopedia. [Online]. Available at: http://www.webopedia.com/
TERM/C/cyber_crime.html (Accessed: Sep 26 2007).

World News (2007) Top 7 Hackers Ever. [Online]. Available at: http://worldandnews.
blogspot.com/2007_04_14_archive.html (Accessed: Sep 26 2007).

Z2Z (2007) Business Glossary. [Online]. Available at: http://www.z2z.com/
cgi-bin/glossary.cgi (Accessed: Sep 26 2007).

ZoneAlarm (2007) ZoneAlarm – Proactive Firewall protection with multiple layers of
security that stop inbound, outbound, and program attacks. [Online]. Available at:
http://www.zonealarm.com/store/content/catalog/products/sku_list_za.jsp?dc=12bms
&ctry=US&lang=en (Accessed: Jul 11 2007).

Zoysa, K.D., Goonatillake, K.S. and Thilakarathna, K.M. (2007) Cybercrime Forensics
Experiences in a Developing Country. Proceedings of the 1st International Confer-
ence on Cybercrime Forensics Education and Training CFET 2007, Canterbury Christ
Church University.

5
Encryption

Dave O'Reilly and Paul Stephens

Encryption is the process of converting data from its plain, legible form into a new form which is unreadable, known as an artefact (or artifact). An artefact may be converted back to a readable form with the use of a 'key', a secret piece of information or data. Techniques for encryption predate the digital age and there are many accounts available in the literature on the history of ciphers, codes and similar cryptographic systems. Until recently, relatively secure methods of encryption were largely restricted to 'official' use by security agencies, but nowadays secure encryption technologies are widely available.

Encryption is a valuable technique. Without encryption many modern internet conveniences, such as buying products online with a credit card, would not be secure; an eavesdropper would be able to capture credit card details directly off the internet. However, encryption is also used by those who wish to keep information confidential for criminal purposes including fraud, child pornography and terrorism. For example, members of the Aum Shinri Kyo (Supreme Truth) cult in Japan used encryption to hide their computer-based records and in 1995 members of the cult were responsible for the death of 12 people by sarin gas poisoning on the Tokyo underground.

Investigating Digital Crime   Edited by Robin Bryant and Sarah Bryant
© 2008 John Wiley & Sons, Ltd

Encryption technologies can be broadly divided into two categories, according to their primary purpose:

- encryption of data for transmission on a network;
- encryption of data for relatively long-term storage.

Obviously, the ideal outcome for a forensic computing investigator in either case is the recovery and examination of the unencrypted data. In this chapter we will consider some of the more common situations in which encryption technologies may be encountered, and, from an investigative perspective, how evidence might be gathered.

Encryption presents two problems to an investigator; first, identifying that something is an encrypted artefact, and secondly, decrypting that artefact. For a more detailed discussion of encryption concepts see Schneier (1996) which covers many technical aspects of encryption and its investigation.

5.1 Keys and passwords

A key is required to decrypt an artefact. It is usually a long sequence of data that an individual is unlikely to be able to recall, and is therefore likely to be stored on a digital device or by some other means.

A password is a shorter key, short enough for an average person to memorise. Passwords can be classified as either weak or strong. A weak password is one that is easier to predict; it could be a known word, or a number sequence linked to the user. For obvious reasons, the use of weak passwords is not to be recommended! If a recognisable word is to be used, it should at least be mis-spelt or include irrelevant punctuation marks. A strong password is not predictable and has no meaning (other than its function as a key). It may contain a mixture of numbers, letters, spaces and punctuation marks, and also tends to be longer than a weak password. Passphrases are also used; predictably these are longer than passwords and can also have weak or strong features.

In some instances it may be possible to decrypt transmitted data without initial access to the key, using 'cracking' or 'brute force' techniques such as password guessing, or by exploiting known weaknesses in the encryption technology. Cracking and brute force are the use of dedicated software to run through a dictionary of words (or combinations of words) in an attempt to uncover the password or phrase by chance. Hence the vulnerability of some weak passwords; a password should not be in any dictionary.

In some cases there may be no key to recover from a suspect as many encryption technologies (such as those used for transmitting data across a network, for example SSL/TLS) use randomly generated session keys which are used for only a short period and then discarded (Dierks, 2006). Contrast this with encryption technologies for storage of data on a hard drive; in order to decrypt the data at some point in the future the key must remain useful for a relatively long period of time.

5.1.1 Key pairs

An important type of encryption for transmission works by generating a pair of keys; a public key and a private key. Each user has a key pair; a public key which is known to others, and a private key known only to the user.

Public–private key pairs are essentially used in the following way:

1. the recipient shares their public key with the sender;

2. they (the sender) use the public key to encrypt the information, producing an artefact;

3. the sender sends the artefact to the recipient;

4. the recipient uses their private key to decrypt the artefact.

Clearly the sender must be certain that the public key received is genuinely from the intended recipient. However, public keys are just that; public. Hence the sender will also include a signature message alongside the private key which can be checked using the public key.

Once the information has been encrypted using the recipient's public key, the resulting artefact cannot be decrypted using the recipient's public key, so for the sender, it is a one-way process; no second chance to check the message sent! Therefore, this form of encryption, though relatively simple in technological terms, is very secure. It is virtually impossible to work out the private key from the public key as they are linked only by a complex mathematical algorithm.

An example of a public-private key pair algorithm

Robin Bryant

Cryptography is the process of converting 'plaintext' (ordinary intelligible text or data) into a form which is unintelligible (encrypted, or what UK legislation calls 'protected'). The encryption process uses an algorithm (a mathematical process, in effect a set of instructions) and a key, or set of keys. The ciphertext can be converted back to its original intelligible form, using the algorithm and a key, but not necessarily the same key. Many of an algorithms used for encryption exploit results and theorems from number theory, a branch of pure mathematics.

For example, plaintext such as 'Regulation of Investigatory Powers' would be encrypted into something like 'Y3*&ft599+0'. The latter phrase could be sent openly to a recipient. Provided the recipient has both knowledge and use of the algorithm and the key(s) he or she should be able to decrypt 'Y3*&ft599+0' back to the plaintext 'Regulation of Investigatory Powers'. Note however, that encryption can be used for any data, not just data representing text. All data, including pictures, videos and audio files are stored in binary format and so are readily converted into numerical form; software encryption packages do this automatically.

Let's take a simple example and suppose that Bob wants to encrypt the message 1 234 and send it to Anneka.

Anneka chooses her encryption method (for example, RSA) and makes Bob aware of this. She then chooses two prime numbers such as 26 863 and 102 001 (a prime number is any number that is not divisible by any whole number other than one and itself).

Next she multiplies these two prime numbers together:

$$26\,863 \times 102\,001 = 2\,740\,052\,863.$$

She follows this by reducing each prime by one, and multiplying the resulting answers:

$$26\,862 \times 102\,000 = 2\,739\,924\,000.$$

Next she needs to choose two other numbers that must have a particular mathematical relationship with the previous result, 2 739 924 000. These two numbers have to be chosen carefully so that:

(a) one of the numbers shares no common divisor (other than 1) with the number 2 739 924 000;

(b) the other number (which also shares no common divisor with 2 739 924 000), when multiplied by the choice made in a) and then divided by 2 739 924 000 leaves a remainder of exactly 1.

By 'trial and error' (in reality a mathematical process called Euclid's Extended Algorithm), Anneka finds two numbers that satisfy the criteria, namely 103 (satisfying part (a)) and 1 143 851 767 (satisfying part (b)).

(To check this, calculate $103 \times 1\,143\,851\,767 = 117\,816\,732\,001$. Then check that 2 739 924 000 goes into this 43 times leaving a remainder of exactly 1. In practice, cryptographic software is used to find these two numbers).

At this stage note that the two numbers 103 and 2 740 052 863 are Anneka's **public key**. (It would probably be more accurate to describe this as Anneka's **public lock**, but the term 'public key' is more commonly used in the literature). We will designate 103 as the first part of the public key and 2 740 052 863 the second part of the public key. She sends both parts of her public key to Bob.

The number 1 143 851 767 (from part (b)) is Anneka's **private key**, and she keeps this to herself.

Bob now sets about encrypting his plaintext message 1 234, to be sent to Anneka.

Using a computer, he first raises 1 234 to the power of the first part of Anneka's public key, 103 (that is $1\,234^{103}$; a very large number), and then divides this result by the second part of her public key, (2 740 052 863) and notes the remainder. The remainder is the encrypted message.

In this case the remainder is 1 063 268 443 and hence the encrypted version of 1 234 that Bob sends to Anneka is 1 063 268 443. Note that Bob has not used any information that is kept secret – he has used Anneka's public key.

Anneka now takes Bob's encrypted message and raises it to the power of her private key, 1 143 851 767, and then divides by the second part of the public key, 2 740 052 863. The remainder in this case is exactly 1 234; Anneka has successfully decrypted Bob's message.

5.1.2 Legislation and keys

Legislation in relation to the regulatory ability of an investigating officer to seize encryption keys (and the requirements of a suspect to surrender encryption keys) varies across the world. In the UK it is currently not an offence for the suspect to refuse to surrender encryption keys. The legislation that would give police officers the powers to seize encryption keys (and make it an offence to refuse to surrender encryption keys) is contained in Part III of the Regulation of Investigatory Powers Act 2000, commonly known as known as RIPA. In June 2007 the UK Government published a draft Investigation of Protected Electronic Information code of practice as a step towards the implementation of part III of RIPA scheduled for October 2007.

Encryption: investigative challenges

Robin Bryant

In traditional symmetric cryptography (used until the mid to late 1970s), a plaintext message was encrypted with a secret key and then sent to a recipient. Provided the recipient knew the secret key and the algorithm used for encryption, then in theory the recipient would be able to decrypt the message. The system had a number of advantages, including relative simplicity (for example, both sender and recipient shared the same key).

For more modern forms of asymmetric encryption, the approach is somewhat different. For example, the popular encryption package PGP uses a number of keys, both public and private. An individual using PGP can share his or her public key with others who may then use that public key to encrypt messages. The encrypted messages are then sent, and can be decrypted by the recipients, each using his or her private key. This may appear contradictory: after all, how can keys **both** be openly shared **and** be used to transmit data in a secure, encrypted fashion? An analogy with 'night safes' is often used to explain how this is possible. Night safes are to be found built into the outside wall of high street banks and are used by employees of local shops and others to deposit cash after business has finished for the day. The safe is unlocked with a key, the money is deposited in the special container (which also prevents access to the safe), and then the safe automatically closes and locks itself. Authorised users of the same night safe are all given identical keys; that is they are public. But each user can only deposit cash, not remove the cash of others.

For criminals, such as paedophiles wishing to distribute child pornography, there are obvious advantages to public key encryption methods. By not using a secret key in the transmission process the danger of compromising the security of the message is significantly reduced. Public key systems can also be used to communicate securely with groups of people rather than on the one-to-one basis needed with earlier 'secret key' encryption. These modern forms of encryption are also based on mathematical number theory (see 5.1.1), particularly 'trap door' mathematics. This is a reference to mathematical algorithms that in practice will only work in one direction. This too, requires some explanation. If two prime numbers are multiplied together then the result is a number with only two factors. For example, $3 \times 5 = 15$ and the number 15 only has two factors (3 and 5, but not 2, 4 or 6 etc.) Hence if a person (or a computer running a program) is given the number 15 to factorise they will, sooner or later, arrive at the conclusion that 15 is made up of 3 and 5 multiplied together, but only those numbers. (In contrast 12, say can be thought of as 2×6 or 3×4). If '15' is the encrypted message then it would not take long to establish that the decrypted message is '3' and '5'. However, what if the encrypted message was '5 369 913 727'? It would take a human being a long time to establish that the message here is '93 239' and '57 593' (and only that message). Unfortunately for investigators, public key encryption is an even more difficult challenge than this relatively simple example, as it involves complex manipulation of the prime numbers (see 5.1.1). Indeed, where the private key is sufficiently strong (in terms of length and choice) simple 'brute force' methods alone are unlikely to succeed in breaking public key encryption. There are methods which stand some chance of breaking these forms of encryption but they are laborious and not guaranteed to yield a result (but are probably still worth trying).

However, there are a number of advantages that investigators may have when encountering forms of encryption used by offenders:

- Encryption requires a significant amount of effort and some skill on behalf of the user. For this reason it is possible that at least some communications or files may have been left unencrypted.

- It is not unknown for suspects to write private keys down and take few (if any) steps to hide the information.

- Under Part III of the Regulation of Investigatory Powers Act 2000 (expected to come into force in October 2007), authorised persons will have the power to serve a 'Section 49 Notice' on a person in control of encrypted information. This obliges him or her to disclose the unencrypted version of the information, where such disclosure is necessary in the interests of national security for the prevention or detection of crime, in the interests of the economic well-being of the UK, or for securing the effective exercise by any public authority of any statutory power or duty. There are also circumstances under which the non-disclosure of the private key itself will be an offence.

5.2 Encrypted hard drives

Encryption of hard disk volumes is a technology that has been used for many years. It is a popular technique for protecting sensitive data, particularly for data stored on laptops as a laptop is more likely to be stolen than a desktop. In fact, some company security policies state that sensitive data stored on laptops should always be stored in encrypted volumes. Encrypted volumes are also widely used on servers used for storing sensitive data. A 'volume' on a hard disk is the name given to a storage area where a single file system resides, and a volume usually resides within a single partition of a hard disk.

Disk encryption technologies are not widely used by non-technical computer users, for a variety of reasons; for example the user must:

- know that disk encryption technology exists;

- have the technical skill to correctly configure the software; and

- be prepared to accept the trade-off between security and convenience that is inherent in using encryption software; it is clearly less convenient for a user to have to enter a decryption password before they can access any of their files.

5.2.1 Disk encryption technologies

There are broadly two types of disk encryption technology; those that encrypt a whole physical drive or partition, and those that create an encrypted volume which is stored as a file in a normal file system.

Whole disk encryption

To view a file using whole disk encryption, a decryption key or password is required as the computer is booting up. The key may be entered at the keyboard as part of the boot process or it may be saved on a USB memory stick or other piece of hardware, which must be inserted as the machine is booting. Once the key has been entered, the encrypted volume is mounted and accessed like any other non-encrypted disk volume. Since the entire volume is encrypted, there will be no single file which can be identified as an encrypted volume. In fact, it can sometimes be difficult to even establish the fact that a partition contains an encrypted volume, because the data in the partition might look like garbage.

Most whole disk encryption technologies will not encrypt the boot volume because otherwise the BIOS would need to be able to decrypt the boot volume in order to boot the operating system. The few whole disk encryption systems which do actually encrypt the operating system partition usually require a small unencrypted partition where the core operating system files reside. In such circumstances, the operating system boots from the unencrypted partition and then the operating system can decrypt the larger encrypted volume where most of the data on the computer is stored. Several encryption systems, such as Windows Vista BitLocker work in this way.

Encrypted volumes

The second type of encrypted storage technology creates a file that contains an encrypted volume stored as a file in a normal file system. The file contains an entire file system, and the drive is typically mounted by software running on the operating system. The user is prompted for their password when they first attempt to mount the drive.

5.2.2 Examples of disk encryption technologies

There are many different disk encryption technologies; extensive lists of encryption software and hardware can be found on various websites (e.g. Wikipedia, 2007a; FDE, 2007). The terms used to describe the various encryption systems may vary, and the names of commercial encryption products reflect this variability. For the purposes of the present discussion, we will examine some of the encryption software technologies which function on the Windows platform.

Microsoft Windows Vista BitLocker

Vista BitLocker is a whole disk encryption system which can encrypt the entire operating system volume. It is included in the Enterprise and Ultimate editions of Vista. There are three modes of operation of BitLocker, two of which require specific hardware known as a trusted platform module (TPM) and a compatible BIOS (Microsoft, 2007a, 2007c, 2007d). A TPM is an additional chip inside the computer and it stores the hard disk encryption key.

BitLocker can work in three different ways:

- the TPM releases the key to the operating system once the integrity of the boot files has been verified, with no user interaction in the boot process; or

- the TPM checks early boot components, and then the user enters a PIN or a USB drive which contains the system startup key; or

- the user must provide the system startup key from a USB drive in order for the system to boot (a TPM is not required).

At the time of writing, Microsoft Windows Vista has only been available for a few months. Therefore, the investigative consequences of the new technologies in Vista have not yet been fully assessed, but it seems that BitLocker is unlikely to present a substantial investigative barrier in the short term (Leyden, 2007; Morris, 2007). There are a number of reasons for this:

- BitLocker is only present in two of the Vista versions (Enterprise and Ultimate).

- In two of its three modes of operation, BitLocker requires specialised hardware and a supporting BIOS, which are not yet widely available.

- If a user wishes to store their BitLocker key on a USB drive, the computer's BIOS must support reading USB drives before the operating system has booted.

- The use of BitLocker poses some risks; if any component of the BitLocker system (system BIOS, TPM, etc.) fail, irretrievable data loss will occur. Therefore system backups become essential which increases the likelihood that unencrypted copies of data will be found, particularly in corporate environments.

- If the system is running, it is possible for an investigator to 'dump' the BitLocker encryption key from the running system; the system may then be safely shut down, and the investigator will be able to access the contents of the hard drive at some point in the future.

- Once the operating system is running, BitLocker does not provide any protection against files being copied from the running system; an investigator will be able to access all files on an machine that is already running, (although EFS (discussed below) can be used to protect sensitive files while the system is running.)

The main use of BitLocker is to prevent data extraction from a physical hard drive acquired by a new user; that new user may well be a police investigator following lawful seizure of a computer. The key issue for investigators will be detecting that BitLocker is in use; before shutting down the computer the investigator must take appropriate action (Hogfly, 2007). If such action is not taken and the computer is turned off, BitLocker protected files will be difficult to access subsequently.

Encrypting File System (EFS)

Microsoft's Encrypting File System (EFS) is available in versions of Windows from Windows 2000 onwards (Wikipedia, 2007b). EFS permits individual files to be encrypted and stored on an NTFS file system transparently to the user who owns the file. Each user has a public–private key pair, generated the first time the user encrypts a file using EFS. This system also uses a third key known as a 'file encryption key', or FEK.

The EFS process (Microsoft, 2007b; Morris, 2007) is summarised below.

- An unencrypted file is created by a user.

- An FEK is generated.

- The file encrypted using the FEK.

- The FEK is also encrypted with the user's public key.

- A header containing the encrypted FEK is added to the encrypted file.

- The file is ready to be stored until required.

- To decrypt the file, the user's private key must be used to decrypt the header and extract the FEK.

- Then the decrypted FEK is used to decrypt the contents of the whole file.

If an investigator needs to decrypt files from a seized computer, software such as Elcomsoft (2007a) or GuidanceSoftware (2007) is available. For Windows 2000, an investigator would not need the suspect's username and password, (unless SYSKEY protection is being used). For Windows XP, 2003 or Vista the suspect's password or the administrator's password is required.

Password cracking software can be used to attempt to recover either the administrator or user passwords (Petri, 2007; Ophcrack, 2007). The EFS recovery software packages referred to above both have the ability to run through a dictionary of passwords, but operate quite slowly, and neither are dedicated password crackers. Therefore it is usually recommended that investigators initially use a dedicated password cracker, and that the results of the password cracking are used subsequently with the EFS recovery software.

Even if it is not possible to decrypt the contents of the file, the file metadata such as the creation, modification and access times are still available. Investigators should also be aware that unencrypted versions of the file may be found by searching unallocated space, temporary folders or system backups.

PGPdisk

PGPdisk, included in PGP Desktop, produces an encrypted volume as a file in the normal file system (PGP, 2007). When PGPdisk is installed, an icon is added to the system tray which allows the user to create new PGPdisk volumes. The encrypted volume is stored in a file with the extension '.pgd'.

In newer versions of PGPdisk the encrypted volume expands as more information is encrypted, from a relatively small initial size up to a configured maximum. However in older versions of PGPdisk, if a 2 Gb PGPdisk encrypted volume is created, the entire 2 Gb is allocated even before any information is actually stored. Therefore these files can be very large, up to several Gbs; of course, encrypted files are not always large, but large files are one feature investigators look for as an identifying feature of PGPdisk encrypted files.

When using PGP to encrypt a volume on a desktop or laptop:

- The user will double click on the file that contains the encrypted volume, which will launch the encryption application.

- The user will be prompted for their password or key, which will cause the decryption and mounting of the hard drive.

- The contents of the encrypted volume will then appear as an additional drive on the computer, (in the same way as a USB memory stick drive appears as an additional drive).

PGPdisk can be enabled to auto-dismount a volume after a certain number of minutes of inactivity on a computer. When this feature is enabled, if an open file is left by a user for just a few minutes, the encrypted volume automatically dismounts.

It is not possible to get the PGPdisk encryption password back from the encrypted volume. Software exists for attempting to crack a PGPdisk encryption password using brute force (Elcomsoft, 2007b), but clearly the success of this technique depends on the user having chosen a weak password.

5.2.3 Investigating encrypted disks

The primary goal of the investigator is to obtain the key in order to decrypt and view the contents of an encrypted volume. The key might be obtained from:

- the suspect directly;
- USB memory sticks or backup digital devices in the suspect's location;
- the suspect's mobile phone or PDA, or pieces of paper in or around the suspect's workstation;
- the live system memory of the suspect's computer; or
- the running system of the suspect's computer (BitLocker startup key).

Traditional, non-technical investigative techniques should always be used to attempt to elicit the key from the suspect. If this is not possible, investigators should remember that the encryption of the data stored on disk is carried out in memory, so the encryption key must be in memory for the duration of time that the encrypted volume is mounted. Therefore, capturing a memory dump of the computer before turning it off may preserve the key, which can be extracted from the memory dump later. The key could then be used to decrypt an encrypted volume, even if it had been auto-dismounted before the investigator had gained access to a suspect's computer.

5.3 Email encryption

Email is now one of the most frequently used modes of communication in the world, and the forensic analysis of email is a standard part of the job for most high tech crime investigators. As some readers will be aware, email can be encrypted. Many email clients support encryption either natively or through an add-on or plug-in. The technical difficulty (to the user) associated with encrypting an email is occasionally a function of the user friendliness of the email client rather than due to any inherent complexity. However, the vast majority of email is not encrypted; many users may not be aware that encryption is possible, or do not perceive the added inconvenience as worthwhile. Clearly, criminals are likely on some occasions to use encrypted emails to communicate details about criminal activities.

5.3.1 Technologies for encrypting email

Numerous technologies are available for encrypting email and the vast majority are based on some form of public-private key cryptographic system (Bradley, 2007). One example of such a system is GPG, (GNU Privacy Guard), an open source replacement for PGP, available for most popular operating systems (GPG, 2007; Wikipedia 2007c). A single use session key is generated and used to encrypt the email message. The recipient's public key is used by the sender to encrypt the session key. The recipient then uses their private key to decrypt the session key, and then uses that key to decrypt the email. GPG can use a number of different encryption techniques, and generates keys with lengths between 768 and 2 048 bits, which are extremely large and practically impossible to crack by brute force using current computing technology. The keys themselves are protected with a passphrase which the user must remember in order to decrypt emails.

5.3.2 Investigating encrypted emails

An encrypted email is structurally identical to a normal email except that the content is a garbled set of characters. Typically an encrypted email is structured as a MIME message with a 'content-type' header value of 'multipart/encrypted'. It is technically infeasible to crack most email encryption. Therefore, traditional investigative techniques must be used to acquire keys and passphrases from the suspect, either directly or indirectly. However, even without being able to decrypt the content of an email, it is still possible to carry out standard header analysis on an encrypted email. The header can reveal the usual information such as sender, recipient and so on, and may be used to establish that two individuals are acquainted. Another point to note is that if there is communication between two parties, some of which is encrypted, some of which is not, the investigator may be able to focus their attention on the times and dates of the encrypted emails, in order to assess any significance.

5.4 VoIP

Skype is a popular example of voice over IP (VoIP) software, used to communicate on a daily basis particularly for international calls (the calls are effectively free if both users are on broadband connections). A purpose made Skype handset is plugged into a USB port on the computer, and calls are 'dialled' using the computer screen.

Skype software must be installed on the computers of both the caller and the recipient of the call. The call and chat history are stored in the user's Skype folder in binary '.dbb' files. Both the call signalling information and the voice data are encrypted for transmission across the network. The call signalling information is only encoded using RC4 but the voice data is strongly encrypted using AES (Fabrice, 2005).

Skype voicemail is an additional service that users can pay to have added to their Skype account. It works in much the same way as conventional voicemail; callers can leave a voice message if the recipient is not online at the time they try to ring. The voicemails are stored on Skype's servers until the user listens to them, but once the listener has heard the voicemail it is removed from the Skype server and stored on the user's PC until the user decides to delete it (Skype, 2007b).

5.4.1 Investigating VoIP

From an investigative point of view, there are a number of relevant factors to consider:

- Is Skype installed, or has Skype ever been installed?

- Have calls taken place? (Call signalling information).

- When did the calls take place and how long did they last? (Call and chat history).

- What is the content of the calls? (Voice data).

- Are any voicemail messages stored on the suspect's computer?

Skype presents a difficult challenge for an investigator due to its deliberate obfuscation and encryption of both file formats and network traffic. Further, the Skype binary itself is resistant to analysis because it is stored encoded on disk and only decodes itself in memory as it is running. It also checks for the presence of some common debugging tools and will not run if they are present (Fabrice, 2005).

Various reviews of Skype have been carried out which provide extensive lists of the files and registry keys created by Skype (Bergstrom 2004; Skype, 2006). These can be used to establish that Skype is currently installed, though as different versions of Skype are released, the file and registry entries may change.

It is possible to determine if Skype has been installed on a PC and has since been removed. This is because file remnants are left behind by the uninstall process. By searching the registry for the word 'Skype', various references to Skype DLLs (Dynamic Link Libraries, a form of common shared code utilised by a number of applications) may be found, even if the application has subsequently been uninstalled. This can give the strong indication that Skype had previously been installed on the computer.

In terms of network investigation, call setup information can be gathered and decoded directly from the network traffic. This can be useful in establishing that two suspects are in contact with each other. Even without being able to decrypt the content of the calls, it is still be possible to prove using the signalling information that two individuals were in communication. It should be possible to further evidence that finding by examining the call history on either or both of the two computers from which the calls were made. The call and chat history are stored in the user's Skype folder in binary '.dbb' files, referred to earlier. Tools are available for extracting chat information from the files (e.g. Paraben, 2007). Very little corroborating information is available concerning the structure of the binary '.dbb' files, but a small amount of information is available on the Skype forums (Skype, 2007a). A hex editor can also be used to extract the contents of Skype chat history, although it is difficult to reconstruct an actual conversation in this way.

Packet sniffing the network traffic produced by Skype can produce some useful information to support an investigation. Both the call signalling information and the voice data are encrypted for transmission across the network, and as the call signalling information is only encoded using RC4, it is possible to retrieve call signalling information from the network traffic. The key can be extracted directly from the UDP packets because the RC4 seed key is generated from the source and destination IP addresses and the packet ID.

It is not possible to decrypt the actual voice data as it is strongly encrypted using AES, and only the sender and the recipient can decrypt it (Fabrice, 2005). If the voice data is required, some form of audio 'tap' must be installed on the PC of the suspect to capture voice data from the sound card before it is encrypted and sent across the network. However, this type of monitoring software will often only capture one side of the conversation.

Finally, if the user has voicemail, it is possible to gather voicemails that the user has already listened to from the voicemail directory on the PC. As the voicemails are derived from stored data, listening to such recorded messages is not technically a wire-tap; there are no Interception of Communication issues, and no application needs to be made to a CSP (Communications Service Provider).

5.5 Wireless local area networks

Wireless local area networks (LANs) are another widely used technology which often employ encryption. The arrangement in a typical small domestic office consists of a laptop with a wireless LAN card and a wireless base station, known as an access point. Larger office networks may consist of a substantial number of access points connected together into a cellular network which can cover a large physical area, throughout which users can roam. Many wi-fi networks are very insecure; any computer with wireless access enabled is likely to reveal information ralating to several other networks in the area.

Wardriving is the technique of searching for wireless networks using wi-fi enabled equipment such as a laptop from a car. (The terms warwalking and warbiking are also used for searchers not based in a car.) Access to these networks does not need to be attempted for it to be classified as wardriving.

Many of these networks simply allow access without any sort of authentication, or notification of the owner. This is partly due to ISPs supplying equipment without any of the security features enabled, although this practice may be beginning to change. Of course, attackers do not simply use their operating system's built in wireless detection capabilities; they employ more sophisticated tools such as Netstumbler (2007), Ministumbler (2007), or Kismet (2007), which provide much more information about the nature of the network being scanned.

Armed with detailed information of the victim's wi-fi set-up an attacker can then set about the 'whacking' in earnest. This can range from merely using some-one else's internet connection (called piggybacking) to eavesdropping, theft and electronic vandalism. In any subsequent crime investigation, the investigator will be led to the IP address of the innocent victim's internet connection, and may be unable to locate the real perpetrator.

In the UK no case law currently exists to ascertain the legality of wardriving. However, apart from checking a wireless LAN for vulnerabilities and drawing the public's attention to the problem, there is no justifiable reason for wardriving; it is an activity with little purpose other than to provide opportunities for illegal activities such as piggybacking.

Covert investigations can take advantage of the fact that wireless networks are frequently easy to access and may be used to intercept communications by suspects. Of course, wiretapping legislation must be properly taken into account in these cases. Alternatively, a criminal could deliberately set up a wireless LAN in an insecure configuration; he or she could then mount a defence based on the fact that the wireless network was insecure, and suggest that it might have been used by a number of unidentified outsiders. Investigators should gather evidence from the PC of the suspect to ensure that this particular scenario cannot be claimed as a defence.

5.5.1 Protecting the security of wireless networks

Frequently, wireless LAN equipment is sold to consumers with a default, insecure configuration, with a view to making it easier for the consumer to install without technical support. In the typical home or home office environment, a user may not always possess the technical skills required to reconfigure the access point to a more secure configuration (by employing encryption or other methods). From a security perspective, one of the important features of wireless networks is that their coverage area may physically extend beyond the limits of the building in which the wireless access point is situated. Therefore a person who is not in the same building as the wireless LAN may be able to use wardriving and access the network if it is not configured correctly.

Several technologies have been used to attempt to make wireless LANs as secure as an equivalent wired network including Network ESSID, MAC address filtering, WEP encryption and WPA/WPA2. These are examined below.

Network ESSID

Extended Service Set Identifier (ESSID) is a code number (a 'network name') identifying a particular network. All access points of a particular network are configured to the same ESSID, and in a default configuration, many access points broadcast their ESSID. Therefore uninvited users of wireless networks can see all available wireless LANs along with their network names, and may choose the one that is most appropriate for them. It is possible to configure access points so they do not broadcast their ESSID, but a user who knows an ESSID would still be able to manually enter it and successfully associate with the access point. Additionally, every time a legitimate user associates with the access point, the ESSID is transmitted in plain text across the wireless network, and an attacker can passively sniff the ESSID for a target network from the air. For these reasons, relying on not broadcasting the ESSID provides only a very low level of security.

MAC address filtering

Most access points can be configured with a set of allowed MAC addresses, and a user with a MAC address which is not in the list will not be able to associate with that access point. Unfortunately, for a novice user, MAC address filtering is relatively difficult to set up and maintain. In addition, it is relatively simple for a more experienced and less scrupulous user to spoof a MAC address, thereby outwitting this particular approach to network security.

WEP

WEP (wired equivalent privacy) encryption uses a key that is configured on the access point and on each client. All the traffic on the network is encrypted using a shared key, so the transmitted data is offered a level of protection, equivalent to the level of protection on an otherwise identical wired network. However, WEP has a number of well documented weaknesses (AirCrack 2007; Fluhrer *et al.*, 2001; Stubblefield *et al.*, 2001), and an attacker can crack WEP encryption by gathering a relatively small amount of data, and acquire a WEP key in only a matter of minutes.

WPA/WPA2

After the serious security weaknesses were discovered in WEP (see above), WPA, (Wi-fi Protected Access) was developed with reference to the IEEE802.11i security standard, (IEEE, 2006). In order to provide an improved alternative to

WEP, WPA was implemented immediately, and it meets most of the IEEE802.11i standard. A refined version of WPA (WPA2) implements all of the mandatory components of IEEE802.11i.

Since 2006, WPA2 must be implemented in any new device sold with Wi-Fi certification (Wi-Fi, 2007a, b). There are no known cryptographic problems with WPA/WPA2, but even when WPA enabled devices are present, there are still a number of factors which can lead to an insecure network, such as:

- The default configuration on the device is either 'no encryption' or 'WEP encryption'. WPA/WPA2 must be chosen as the encryption technique on the access point.

- The use of weak passwords. WPA/WPA2 security is heavily dependent on a choice of a strong passphrase, and users are notoriously poor at choosing strong passphrases. Dedicated cracking tools are available to attempt to crack WPA pre-shared keys/passphrases (coWPAtty, 2007). This weakness can be mitigated in a corporate environment by using some of the more advanced features of WPA/WPA2, see below.

Other LAN encryption technologies

In corporate environments, maintaining keys and/or passphrases on every single access point throughout a network is infeasible. Therefore, a number of technologies have been developed to centralise authentication information. Most of these are based on the use of WPA/WPA2 and the Extensible Authentication Protocol (EAP) (RFC 2004). When a user tries to associate with an access point, the access point verifies the user's credentials with a central authentication server. In order to gain access to such a network, authentication credentials must be created on the centralised server.

5.6 Encryption and investigation

In this chapter we have attempted to provide some examples of the situations in which encryption technologies may be encountered and some investigative techniques which can be used in those cases. Common technologies such as hard disk, email, Skype and wireless LAN encryption have been provided as examples of such situations. Encryption presents substantial challenges to the investigator. Currently encryption technologies are not widely used by non-technical users because of the technical barriers and the added inconvenience. It would be naive to assume that this will always remain the case, so procedures and techniques of investigation must be sensitive to the issues pertinent to encrypted artefacts. First responders, forensic investigators and legal professionals all need to be aware of encryption technology and how to identify if it is likely to have been used and how to act in those cases.

Questions

Robin Bryant & Sarah Bryant

1. How prevalent is the use of encryption in criminal activity?

2. What are the weaknesses with symmetric encryption approaches?

3. What are the problems that encryption can cause for an investigation into a digital crime?

4. What are 'digital signatures'?

5. Tom wants to send a message to Alex. Tom and Alex each have a public-private key pair. Which one of these four keys will (a) Tom need to encrypt a message to send to Alex and (b) which key will Alex need to decode the message?

6. In simple terms, how does a 'brute force' password cracker work?

7. What is a 'Section 49 notice' ?

8. What sort of information may be gleaned about a suspect's Skype communications from his or her PC?

9. A concerned home PC user with a wireless network ensures that the ESSID is not broadcast. What level of protection does this afford against unauthorised use of the network?

10. Suggest two reasons why a wireless network might still be insecure, despite the fact that all the hardware employed is WPA2 implemented.

References

AirCrack (2007) aircrack-ptw. [Online]. Available at: http://www.cdc.informatik. tu-darmstadt.de/aircrack-ptw/ (Accessed: Oct 10 2007).

Bergstrom, D. (2004) An analysis of Skype VoIP application for use in a corporate environment. [Online]. Available at: http://www.geocities.com/bergstromdennis/ Skype_Analysis_1_3.pdf (Accessed: Oct 10 2007).

Bradley, T. (2007) Why you should encrypt your email. [Online]. Available at: http:// netsecurity.about.com/cs/emailsecurity/a/aa051004.htm (Accessed: Oct 10 2007).

coWPAtty (2007) coWPAtty MAIN. [Online]. Available at: http://www. wirelessdefence.org/Contents/coWPAttyMain.htm (Accessed: Oct 10 2007).

Dierks, T. (2006) The transport layer security (tls) protocol. [Online]. Available at: http://tools.ietf.org/html/rfc434624 (Accessed: Oct 10 2007).

Elcomsoft (2007a) Elcomsoft: Advanced efs data recovery. [Online]. Available at: http://www.elcomsoft.com/aefsdr.html (Accessed: Oct 10 2007).

Elcomsoft (2007b) Password recovery software. [Online]. Available at: http://www. elcomsoft.com/prs.html (Accessed: Oct 10 2007).

Fabrice, D. (2005) Skype uncovered: Security study of Skype. [Online]. Available at: http://www.ossir.org/windows/supports/2005/2005–11–07/EADS-CCR_Fabrice_ Skype.pdf (Accessed: Oct 10 2007).

FDE (2007) Full disk encryption providers. [Online]. Available at: http://www.full-disk-encryption.net/Full_Disc_Encryption.html (Accessed: Oct 10 2007).

Fluhrer, S., Mantin, I. and Shamir, A. (2001) Weaknesses in the key scheduling algorithm of RC4. Eighth Annual Workshop on Selected Areas in Cryptography, Toronto, Ontario, Canada, Aug 16–17, 2001.

GPG (2007) The Gnu privacy guard. [Online]. Available at: http://www.gnupg.org (Accessed: Oct 10 2007).

GuidanceSoftware (2007) Encase forensic modules. [Online]. Available at: http:// www.guidancesoftware.com/products/ef_modules.aspx (Accessed: Oct 10 2007).

Hogfly (2007) Detecting bitlocker. [Online]. Available at: http://forensicir.blogspot.com/ 2007/03/detecting-bitlocker.html (Accessed: Oct 10 2007).

IEEE (2006) Get IEEE 802®. IEEE Standards Association [Online]. Available at: http://standards.ieee.org/getieee802/download/802.11i-2004.pdf (Accessed: Oct 12 2007).

Kismet (2007) Kismet-2007–01-R1b. [Online]. Available at: http://www.kismetwireless. net/code/kismet-2007–01-R1b.tar.gz (Accessed: Aug 1 2007).

Leyden, J. (2007) Vista encryption 'no threat' to computer forensics. [Online]. Available at: http://www.theregister.co.uk/2007/02/02/computer_forensics_vista/ (Accessed: Oct 10 2007).

Microsoft (2007a) Bitlocker drive encryption. [Online]. Available at: http://technet. microsoft.com/en-us/windowsvista/aa905065.aspx (Accessed: Oct 10 2007).

Microsoft (2007b) How efs works. [Online]. Available at: http://www.microsoft.com/

technet/prodtechnol/windows2000serv/reskit/distrib/dsck_efs_duwf.mspx (Accessed: Oct 10 2007).

Microsoft (2007c) Windows BitLocker drive encryption frequently asked questions. [Online]. Available at: http://technet2.microsoft.com/WindowsVista/en/library/58358421-a7f5-4c97-ab41–2bcc61a58a701033.mspx (Accessed: Oct 10 2007).

Microsoft (2007d) Windows BitLocker drive encryption step-by-step guide. [Online]. Available at: http://technet2.microsoft.com/WindowsVista/en/library/c61f2a12–8ae6–4957-b031-97b4d762cf311033.mspx (Accessed: Oct 10 2007).

Ministumbler (2007) MiniStumbler 0.4.0 Installer. [Online]. Available at: http://downloads.netstumbler.com/downloads/ministumblerinstaller_0_4_0.exe (Accessed: Aug 1 2007).

Morris, J. (2007) Notes on Vista forensics, part one. [Online]. Available at: http://www.securityfocus.com/infocus/1889/ (Accessed: Oct 10 2007).

Netstumbler (2007) NetStumbler 0.4.0 Installer. [Online]. Available at: http://downloads.netstumbler.com/downloads/netstumblerinstaller_0_4_0.exe (Accessed: Aug 1 2007).

Ophcrack (2007) Ophcrack. [Online]. Available at: http://ophcrack.sourceforge.net/ (Accessed: Oct 10 2007).

Paraben (2007) Chat examiner. [Online]. Available at: http://www.paraben-forensics.com/catalog/product_info.php?cPath=25&products_id=162 (Accessed: Oct 10 2007).

Petri, D. (2007) How can I gain access to a Windows NT/2000/XP/2003 computer if I forgot the administrator's password? How can I reset the administrator's password if I forgot it? [Online]. Available at: http://www.petri.co.il/forgot_administrator_password.htm (Accessed: Oct 10 2007).

PGP (2007) PGP Desktop Home. [Online]. Available at: http://www.pgp.com/products/desktop_home/index.html (Accessed: Oct 10 2007).

RFC (2004) Extensible authentication protocol. [Online]. Available at: http://tools.ietf.org/html/rfc3748 (Accessed: Oct 10 2007).

RIPA (2007) Regulation of Investigatory Powers Act. Home Office Security [Online]. Available at: http://security.homeoffice.gov.uk/ripa/ (Accessed: Oct 12 2007).

Schneier, B. (1996) *Applied Cryptography*. Chichester: Wiley.

Skype (2006) Skype guide for network administrators. [Online]. Available at: http://www.skype.com/security/guide-for-network-admins.pdf (Accessed: Oct 10 2007).

Skype (2007a) Export/reading of chat archives, can I export and read the chat archives? [Online]. Available at: http://forum.skype.com/index.php?s=4fc612820f7fb80f4ff47fdec301f780&showtopic=77213 (Accessed: Oct 10 2007).

Skype (2007b) Voicemail Beta Test Frequently Asked Questions. [Online]. Available at: http://www.skype.com/help/faq/voicemail.html (Accessed: Oct 10 2007).

Stubblefield, A., Ioannidis, J. and Rubin, A.V. (2001) Using the Fluhrer, Mantin and Shamir attack to break WEP. [Online]. Available at: http://www.isoc.org/isoc/conferences/ndss/02/proceedings/papers/stubbl.pdf (Accessed: Oct 10 2007).

Wi-Fi (2007a) WPA knowledge centre. [Online]. Available at: http://www.Wi-Fi.org/knowledge_center/wpa (Accessed: Oct 10 2007).

Wi-Fi (2007b) WPA2 knowledge centre. [Online]. Available at: http://www.Wi-Fi.org/knowledge_center/wpa2 (Accessed: Oct 10 2007).

Wikipedia (2007a) Comparison of disk encryption software. [Online]. Available at: http://en.wikipedia.org/wiki/Comparison of disk encryption software (Accessed: Oct 10 2007).

Wikipedia (2007b) Encrypting file system. [Online]. Available at: http://en.wikipedia.org/wiki/Encrypting_File_System (Accessed: Oct 12 2007).

Wikipedia (2007c) Gnu privacy guard. [Online]. Available at: http://en.wikipedia.org/wiki/Gpg (Accessed: Oct 10 2007).

6

IPR and Technological Protection Measures

Paul Stephens

Intellectual property rights (IPR) is a general term encompassing the privileges accorded to the creators and owners of creative work (intellectual property, or IP) including inventions, designs, software, music, films, and written works. Creators or owners with IPR are afforded exclusive rights concerning the reproduction and use of the work. It has been suggested that creativity and innovation will be encouraged if creators and owners are able to profit from their work whilst at the same time making it available to the public (UK Intellectual Property Office, 2007).

In the UK, an IPR is achieved through five means:

- copyright – economic rights over material such as music;

- designs – appearance of a product e.g. a type of Nike trainer;

- patents – a new invention that usually has to be 'industrially applicable';

- trade marks – a sign that distinguishes a company e.g. the McDonald's logo.

- other means - for example, plant breeders' rights

Investigating Digital Crime   Edited by Robin Bryant and Sarah Bryant
© 2008 John Wiley & Sons, Ltd

Digital transgressions of IPR usually involve the infringement of copyright. The legislation covering IPR and copyright is complex, and is contained in several Acts and other pieces of legislation, as shown in figure 6.1.

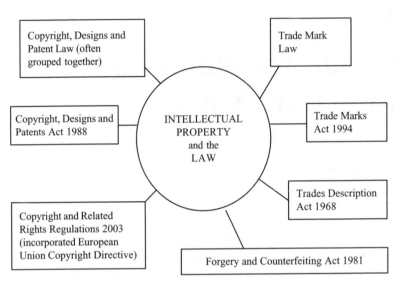

Figure 6.1   Legislation relating to IPR and copyright

6.1 Copyright

Copyright applies to all forms of artistic work, such as literature, computer programs, art, and audio and visual recordings, and automatically comes into force as soon as a work is created by any person; no registration process is required. The copyright holder maintains a legal right to charge for copying, adapting, distributing, renting, lending or performing the work. Usually copyrighted work can only be reproduced and used with the holder's permission, but there are exceptions to this, such as limited use for non-commercial research or personal study. If copyright is breached, the holder has a legal right to seek both an injunction to stop the breach of copyright and to seek appropriate compensation, and the copyright holder can also claim any unauthorised copies of the work. With the widespread use of digital technology and the internet, copyright infringement of digital work has become technically simpler and less expensive to enact.

6.1.1 Digital rights management

Digital rights management (DRM) encompasses a range of technologies that creators or owners may use in an attempt to protect the copyright of digital works. It places restrictions on the ways a consumer may use a digital work. The copying of a work may be completely prohibited or alternatively limited to a set number; the devices on which content may be used can also be specified. Copyright holders applying DRM techniques, such as large sections of the music and film industries, claim that DRM is necessary to help eliminate piracy, to protect the rights of content producers and to maintain low costs for consumers. Opponents of DRM, such as the Electronic Frontier Foundation (EFF), claim that such measures do nothing to prevent widespread copyright infringement on a commercial scale, whilst at the same time DRM interferes with consumers' legitimate use of content (EFF, 2007).

The Free Software Foundation (FSF) is one of the major critics of DRM, and claim that the term digital rights management is '... misleading, since it refers to systems that are designed to take away and limit your rights. So, we suggest you use the term "Digital Restrictions Management" instead.' (FSF, 2007a). FSF have set up a campaign, 'DefectiveByDesign.org' (2007a), which claims that 'DRM products have features built-in that restrict what jobs they can do. These products have been intentionally disabled from the users' perspective, and are therefore 'defective by design' (DefectiveByDesign.org, 2007b). From the perspective of artists, studios, producers and distributors however, it could be argued that consumer expectations are unrealistic.

Photocopiers, tape recorders, CD and DVD burners, mp3 rippers and the 'cut and paste' function on home computers have been widely available for a number of years, enabling consumers to copy and distribute copyright-protected content. Many consumers appear to be unconcerned (if not unaware) that this practice is illegal. Recent attempts to restrict such activities have caused some resentment amongst more active consumers, who argue that fair use of the digital content should include the right to make copies for their own use, and using any device. To some extent the House of Commons Select Committee on Culture, Media and Sport echoes this opinion, concluding in its recent report that

> ... the Government should draw up a new exemption permitting copying within domestic premises for domestic use (including portable devices such as MP3 players, and vehicles owned or used regularly by the household) but not onward transmission of copied material. (Great Britain. Culture, Media and Sport Select Committee, 2007).

The committee also criticised the current application of DRM, stating that consumers have been treated unfairly and that on occasions DRM had contravened exemptions to UK copyright laws. It recommended that DRM is used with care, and that for consumers purchasing protected media, the restrictions on the use of the media should be made clearer.

6.2 IPR in practice

The following section examines some specific approaches to the protection of intellectual property.

6.2.1 Software activation

Microsoft is one of the biggest producers of proprietary software for the personal computer; their range of Windows operating systems is one of the most popular in the world, and Microsoft Office has also sold well. In 1976, the founder of Microsoft, William Henry (Bill) Gates, wrote an open letter to 'hobbyists' (users of BASIC computer software at the time; for example, members of California's Homebrew Computer Club) suggesting that 'most of you steal your software' (Digibarn.com, 2007). This was effectively the beginning of a protracted effort on the part of Microsoft and others to protect their IPR. Microsoft's more recent attempts to restrict the use of their software include Product Keys, Product Activation and Windows Genuine Advantage.

In the early days of the PC, software was distributed on disks that could be easily copied, and the copies usually contained a full and unencumbered version of the software. To try to prevent this kind of IP theft, a modified system was introduced; additional information was required in order to install and use a full working copy of the software. The additional information was often a product key, usually consisting of a unique series of numbers and/or letters, linked by a mathematical algorithm to the software. However, the same key could be used to activate any number of copies of the software; unsurprisingly, the key was distributed along with illegal copies of the software. With the dramatic expansion of the internet, images of the software disks and the product keys could be posted on a single site. As download speeds increased, the practice of using product keys became less effective for the companies concerned and large software manufacturers such as Microsoft sought a more secure alternative.

6.2.2 Product activation

A common form of software IP protection is 'product activation'. After purchasing new software, the consumer has to contact the manufacturer and quote an 'activation identifier', computed from the hardware of a computer and the product key of the newly purchased software. The manufacture checks that the key (and therefore that copy of the software) has not been used previously. On verification of the licence, the manufacturer sends an 'installation ID' to the consumer, who can then use it to activate the software.

Windows XP, released in 2001, was the first Microsoft product to use Product Activation. However, whilst still in Beta testing, The Register reported that Windows XP Product Activation was '...full of gaping holes, and can be fooled almost completely' (Lettice, 2001). These fears appeared to be borne out when only days after the release, reports emerged that Windows XP was anything but tamper-proof, and that pirate copies could be easily bought in Asia (BBC, 2001). Although Microsoft continues to update and improve its activation procedures with the release of Vista, recently developed techniques such as the Vista BIOS attack (Clarke, 2007) can circumvent security features.

6.2.3 Installation of monitoring software

This particular monitoring software is installed on a consumer's computer, enabling a user to verify whether a particular piece of software is legitimate on a particular computer (Microsoft, 2007a). It checks the authenticity of the operating system in a similar way to product activation systems. Microsoft introduced this type of system, 'Windows Genuine Advantage' (WGA), and claims that 'Every day Windows Genuine Advantage helps customers all over the world who are victims of software piracy get genuine.' (Microsoft, 2007b). Critics such as Rasch (2006), however, claim that this is anything but a consumer protection programme. Rather, he claims it is a heavy-handed, perhaps even an illegal way, of Microsoft and other software manufacturers attempting to protect their intellectual property. He explains that consumers who wish to keep up to date with the latest software patches and security updates are forced to install WGA, and that it works in a similar way to some kinds of spyware, and is therefore at least unethical if not illegal. Furthermore, the identification of a particular piece of software as an illegal copy confers no real advantage to the consumer.

6.2.4 Embedded restrictions

On-line music stores have proved to be very popular amongst users of all ages. Prompted by requests from the music industry that artists' IP should be protected, systems have been developed that embed restrictions into the downloaded music files. The downloaded files can be played back, but only on a limited range and number of devices. One example of such a system is Fairplay developed by Apple for use with iPods.

One way of circumventing Fairplay was to burn the downloaded tracks to CD and then to use a ripper to create mp3s. Whilst the burning of tracks to CD is legal under the scheme, converting them, and thus removing the electronic restrictions, is (at best) a legally grey area. This method of sidestepping the FairPlay protection can be fairly time consuming and so quicker methods have been developed, such as QTFairUse (BBC, 2006).

Current developments may make these attempts at defeating FairPlay unnecessary. In February 2007, Steve Jobs (co-founder of Apple) issued an open letter to the music industry calling on them to abandon DRM (Jobs, 2007). In the release, he claimed that DRM was ineffective against piracy and an annoyance to legitimate consumers. He strongly suggested dispensing with DRM and asked his readers to

> Imagine a world where every online store sells DRM-free music encoded in open licensable formats. In such a world, any player can play music purchased from any store, and any store can sell music which is playable on all players. This is clearly the best alternative for consumers, and Apple would embrace it in a heartbeat (Jobs, 2007).

Some commentators treated this proposal with scepticism (e.g. Thomson, 2007); however, in April 2007, Apple announced that EMI tracks sold by the company would be available with and without DRM protection. Although the price of unprotected tracks is slightly higher (99 pence compared with 79 pence for protected tracks) the quality is higher (256 kbps, compared with 128 kbps). It has since emerged that downloaded tracks also contain information about the purchaser (BBC, 2007); this data could be used to identify those who share or sell music illegally. Concerns have been raised that the data could be easily manipulated to implicate an innocent person of music piracy.

6.2.5 Malicious software on music CDs

Sony BMG is one of the largest music companies in the world, and much of the revenue for Sony BMG is derived from the lucrative CD market. CDs are unprotected by DRM technology; CD players were developed before such copy protection measures were invented. More recently, CD-RW drives, mp3 ripping and basic home computers have greatly facilitated the copying of CDs.

In an attempt to target this kind of piracy, Sony BMG introduced new copy protection measures on music CDs. In 2005, Mark Russinovich, an employee of Microsoft and well-known technical author, published an article as part of his blog, 'Sony, Rootkits and Digital Rights Management Gone Too Far' (Russinovich, 2005). Russinovich outlined how following the results of a scan he had conducted while testing a new version of RootkitRevealer he had discovered that a Sony BMG CD he had purchased had installed a 'rootkit' on his machine. A rootkit is a piece of malicious software (malware) that is often used by criminal hackers to hide the installation of any files and other system details that should not be present on a victim's computer. Russinovich goes on to state how the software was poorly implemented, the end user licence agreement (EULA) did not make the nature of the installation of the application clear, and that the malware secretly used system resources such as his CPU. He also showed how difficult it was for a user to delete the software without undermining the stability of his or her system. The software found by Russinovich was a DRM solution called Extended Copy Protection (XCP) and another copy protection technology used by Sony BMG, MediaMax Technology, was also later found to contain similar malicious aspects.

Following the publication of Russinovitch's article and intense media interest, several lawsuits were filed against Sony BMG; XCP and MediaMax were withdrawn from use and software removal tools were suddenly made available. Millions of CDs were also recalled and replaced, and compensation payments were made to many consumers affected by the malware.

Seeking to recoup millions of dollars in lost revenue, Sony BMG has since filed a lawsuit against the designers of the MediaMax Technology, claiming that the software was defective and that the designers should provide compensation for losses incurred. The designers, Amergence, however argue that the software was based on Sony BMG's specifications (OUT-LAW News, 2007).

At the time of writing, no major record labels are advertising new CD protection schemes. However, in the cases against Sony BMG, whilst the courts ruled that

Sony BMG must label the CDs appropriately for the next 12 months (Orlowski, 2006), no ruling specifically prohibited the use of CD protection schemes in the future.

6.2.6 The film industry

Compared with the music industry, the film industry seems to have adopted technological protection measures more effectively. Generally, the protection procedures are similar to those used by Apple in the music industry: both the media and players are in some way controlled. However, unlike the music industry, the technology for protection procedures in the film industry is available to all film studios and suppliers. This is a major advantage for the industry; international trade in illegally copied films is complicated by the division of the global market into regions, each with its own content scrambling system (CSS) for encrypting DVDs. To play back a decrypted version of the DVD, a DVD player from the corresponding region is required, and so producing usable copies of films is less straightforward; different copies are needed for different regions. Despite this, controlling movie piracy remains a major challenge for both the industries concerned and law enforcement agencies.

DeCSS was one of the most well-publicised breaches of film protection measures. First released in 1999, DeCSS is a computer program that decrypts CCS encoded DVDs. Once decrypted, any regional restrictions can be lifted, compulsory trailers and/or warnings can be bypassed, and most significantly, the DVD can be easily copied. One of the DeCCS developers claimed that his intention was to allow DVDs to be watched under the Linux operating system, and that DeCCS was only released on Windows for 'testing' purposes, (because at the time the file system support for DVDs under Linux was still in development (Slashdot, 2004)). Despite his claim, the movie industry attempted to prosecute the individual concerned, but he was acquitted of all charges (BBC, 2004).

Following the cracking of CSS, film distributors sought other ways to protect their content (such as ARccOS), however much of the focus has been on trying to prevent the distribution of DVD copying programs similar to DeCSS. With the advent of new formats such as Blu-ray and HD-DVD, new and more secure copyright encryption techniques have been deployed. However, it has been reported that the schemes used by these newer formats have already been cracked, (Leydon, 2007).

6.3 Open source alternatives

The techniques used to protect IP in digital formats have in a number of cases failed to stop the illegal reproduction and use of electronic content. There are undoubtedly many complex reasons for this; however part of the explanation must surely be the significant profits to be made by circumventing technical copyright protection measures. Many of the measures used by companies have simply turned out to be flawed, sometimes in ethical as well as in technological terms. Accusations of overcharging, misinformation, and invasion of privacy have in many cases been justifiable, however it is generally accepted that the owners of creative work should have the right to protect their intellectual property.

Selling digital media without embedded restrictions might provide a workable solution, however other, more radical alternatives could also be considered. Open source (OSI, 2007) and free software (FSF, 2007b), Creative Commons licenses (CC, 2007) and Web 2.0 technologies such as YouTube (2007) have all been used to successfully make money without technological restrictions being placed upon consumers.

Questions

Robin Bryant & Sarah Bryant

1. How ubiquitous is 'piracy' as a cultural practice, beyond music filesharing?

2. What role do 'amateur' IPR infringements (such as public use of P2P) play in the development of IPR crime?

3. What is the evidence for the existence of links between IPR crime and other forms of criminality (for example, terrorism)?

4. To what extent is the increased use of digital technologies contributing to the development of IPR crime?

5. What arguments support the assertion that the response to music piracy is, at least in part, a form of labelling? How convinced are you by these arguments?

6. Why is there renewed interest in 'binary newsgroups'?

7. Your friend purchases a new photo editing program and installs it from the CD. The results are excellent. How does product activation prevent the use of the program disc on your PC?

References

BBC (2001) Pirates target Windows XP. BBC News [Online]. Available at: http://news. bbc.co.uk/1/hi/sci/tech/1633875.stm (Accessed: Aug 8 2007).

BBC (2004) Film firms lose DVD piracy battle. BBC News [Online]. Available at: http:// news.bbc.co.uk/1/hi/technology/3371975.stm (Accessed: Aug 9 2007).

BBC (2006) iTunes copy protection 'cracked'. BBC News [Online]. Available at: http:// news.bbc.co.uk/1/hi/6083110.stm (Accessed: Aug 9 2007).

BBC (2007) 'Personal data' in iTunes tracks. BBC News [Online]. Available at: http:// news.bbc.co.uk/1/hi/technology/6711215.stm (Accessed: Aug 8 2007).

CC (2007) Creative Commons. [Online]. Available at: http://creativecommons.org/ (Accessed: Aug 8 2007).

Clarke, G. (2007) Microsoft 'wait-and-see' on Vista BIOS hack. [Online]. Available at: http://www.theregister.co.uk/2007/04/11/vista_oem_product_activation/ (Accessed: Aug 8 2007).

DefectiveByDesign.org (2007a) The Campaign to Eliminate DRM. [Online]. Available at: http://www.fsf.org/campaigns/drm.html (Accessed: Aug 7 2007).

DefectiveByDesign.org (2007b) About DefectiveByDesign. [Online]. Available at: http://defectivebydesign.org/about (Accessed: Aug 7 2007).

Digibarn. Com (2007) An Open Letter to Hobbyists February 3 1976. [Online]. Available at: http://www.digibarn.com/collections/newsletters/homebrew/V2_01/homebrew _V2_01_p2.jpg (Accessed: Oct 10 2007)

EFF (2007) Digital Rights Management and Copy Protection Schemes. [Online]. Available at: http://www.eff.org/IP/DRM/ (Accessed: Aug 7 2007).

FSF (2007a) Digital Restrictions Management and Treacherous Computing. [Online]. Available at: http://www.fsf.org/campaigns/drm.html (Accessed: Aug 7 2007).

FSF (2007b) FSF – The Free Software Foundation. [Online]. Available at: http://www. fsf.org/ (Accessed: Aug 10 2007).

Great Britain. Culture, Media and Sport Select Committee (2007) Culture, Media and Sport – Fifth Report. [Online]. Available at: http://www.publications.parliament. uk/pa/cm200607/cmselect/cmcumeds/509/50902.htm (Accessed: Aug 7 2007).

Jobs, S. (2007) Thoughts on Music. [Online]. Available at: http://www.apple.com/ hotnews/thoughtsonmusic/ (Accessed: Aug 8 2007).

Lettice, J. (2001) WinXP product activation cracked: totally, horribly, fatally. [Online]. Available at: http://www.theregister.co.uk/2001/07/23/winxp_product_ activation_cracked_totally/ (Accessed: Aug 8 2007).

Leydon, J. (2007) Latest AACS crack 'beyond revocation'. [Online]. Available at: http://www.theregister.co.uk/2007/05/04/aacs_crack/ (Accessed: Aug 9 2007).

Microsoft (2007a) Microsoft Genuine Advantage Program Information. [Online]. Available at: http://www.microsoft.com/genuine/ProgramInfo.aspx?displaylang= en&sGuid=6aeaea54-fdfb-494e-aaf2-cf7be3293c88 (Accessed: Aug 8 2007).

Microsoft (2007b) Genuine Microsoft Software. [Online]. Available at: http://www.microsoft.com/genuine/default.aspx (Accessed: Aug 8 2007).

Orlowski (2006) How fat is my DRM. [Online]. Available at: http://www.theregister.co.uk/2006/12/20/sony_rootkit_drm_settlement/ (Accessed: Aug 9 2007).

OSI (2007) Home – Open Source Initiative. [Online]. Available at: http://www.opensource.org/ (Accessed: Aug 9 2007).

OUT-LAW News (2007) Sony BMG sues DRM developer. [Online]. Available at: http://www.out-law.com/default.aspx?page=8286 (Accessed: Aug 9 2007).

Rasch, M. (2006) Windows Genuine Disadvantage. [Online]. Available at: http://www.securityfocus.com/columnists/409 (Accessed: Aug 8 2007).

Russinovitch, M. (2005) Sony, Rootkits and Digital Rights Management Gone Too Far. [Online]. Available at: http://blogs.technet.com/markrussinovich/archive/2005/10/31/sony-rootkits-and-digital-rights-management-gone-too-far.aspx (Accessed: Aug 9 2007).

Slashdot (2004) Jon Johansen's Answers to Your DeCSS Questions. [Online]. Available at: http://slashdot.org/interviews/00/02/04/1133241.shtml (Accessed: Aug 9 2007).

Thompson, B. (2007) 'Why I don't believe Steve Jobs'. [Online]. Available at: http://news.bbc.co.uk/1/hi/technology/6353889.stm (Accessed: Aug 8 2007).

UK Intellectual Property Office (2007) UK Intellectual Property Office for creativity and innovation. [Online]. Available at: http://www.ipo.gov.uk/ (Accessed: Aug 7 2007).

YouTube (2007) YouTube – Broadcast Yourself. [Online]. Available at: http://www.youtube.com/ (Accessed: Aug 10 2007).

7

Plastic Card Crime

Robin Bryant and Paul Stephens

Physical objects such as keys have been used for centuries as a means of implementing security and controlling access. One digital equivalent of the key is the plastic card, widely used for financial purposes, membership cards, digital television access cards and a plethora of customer loyalty cards.

7.1 Plastic cards

There are two main types of plastic card in use today:

- the traditional magnetic swipe card (becoming less common in the UK); and

- the smart card, with an embedded electronic chip (more recently introduced).

Many plastic cards also have both a magnetic stripe and a chip, although generally the magnetic stripe is only used when circumstances dictate (so-called 'fallback'), such as a failure of the chip and terminal to communicate. These cards all have some means of recording the identity and entitlements of the cardholder.

Investigating Digital Crime   Edited by Robin Bryant and Sarah Bryant
© 2008 John Wiley & Sons, Ltd

7.1.1 Swipe cards

Swipe cards can be read from, and written to, but little else. In this sense they are 'dumb'. The information is stored in a magnetic stripe, sometimes erroneously referred to as a magnetic strip. They are only usually written to once; the information stored on the card is not usually altered once the card has been issued to the user.

There are normally three tracks in parallel within a single magnetic stripe, and the individual tracks are not visible. Data is stored digitally within a track; each track is divided into 'domains', each containing magnetic particles. If the magnetic flux is reversed within a domain this indicates a 'one'. If there is no flux reversal, this indicates a 'zero'.

The portion of track shown below is storing the data 0 1 1 0 0 1 0 1.

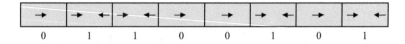

Figure 7.1   How data is stored on a magnetic stripe

The first and second tracks are most frequently used to record the relevant data; the third track does not usually contain any meaningful data. Details of the second track are shown in figure 7.2.

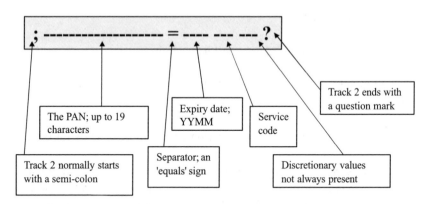

Figure 7.2   Track two contains up to 37 numeric characters

7.1.2 Smart cards

Smart cards resemble miniature computers – they can be written to, be read and can perform various computational functions. This is what makes them 'smart'.

There is a broad distinction between smart cards which are 'memory cards' and others which are 'chip cards'.

Memory cards store information on a type of rewriteable memory called EEPROM which uses transistors. One example of a memory card is the familiar phone card which can be used in public pay phones; the memory is rewritten each time the card is used, recording the time or credit left on the card.

Chip cards are more sophisticated (and hence more expensive to manufacture), and contain a microprocessor chip that includes ROM and RAM as well as EEPROM. Examples of chip cards include many debit and credit cards, and SIM cards for mobile phones. Smart cards also can be used as part of a procedure for controlling access to a facility or service. An example of the latter application is to control access to a pay-TV service, transmitted terrestrially, by cable or satellite.

Figure 7.3 shows the contacts to the chip on a smart card. These can be clearly seen on any smart card, and are commonly referred to as the chip. However the chip itself is normally underneath the contacts and is embedded within the card; only the contacts are visible. There is an accepted standard for the positions of contacts and their functions (as defined by ISO 7816-2).

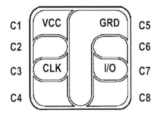

Figure 7.3 Chip contacts on a smart card

The contacts on the chip make electrical contact with the interior of a card reader.

- C1 connects the chip to the power provided by the card reader.

- C2 is the connection for a reset signal from the card reader.

- C3 is the connection for a clock signal, to record on the chip the time and date the card was used.

- C7 is the input and output connection between the chip and the card reader. (For credit and debit cards, the amount for each transaction, and whether the payment was made on or offline may be recorded by the chip).

• C5 is the electrical earthing connection for the card and the card reader.

The contacts C4, C6 and C8 are not in use for this particular module.

7.1.3 Satellite TV cards

Companies seeking to protect access to their subscription TV services frequently use a system involving a chip card and a conditional access module (CAM) built into the receiver. In many cases, the chip in the card is married to the specific CAM in a particular receiver. Once a subscription has been paid, a satellite TV provider will 'unlock' various services (such as particular film or sports channel) by sending a signal to the subscriber's receiver. The signal is usually transmitted by the satellite, and although it is received by all receivers, only the subscriber's particular receiver responds, due to its unique CAM and smart card configuration. Alternatively, the signal may be sent directly through the subscriber's phone line to a modem inside the satellite receiver. For obvious reasons, signals containing data from the chip on the smart card are not transmitted in a plain format but are instead encrypted. This encrypted message will be combined with unique information from the card and CAM and, provided the 'trap door' mathematical algorithm is satisfied (see 5.1.2), the settings within a receiver will be changed – for example, permitting access to a particular TV channel, or suite of channels.

7.1.4 Credit and debit cards

Plastic cards for purchasing goods and taking money from a cash-point (automatic teller machine or ATM) may be swipe cards or smart chip cards, or a combination of the two. The main features of this type of card are shown in figure 7.4. Credit and debit cards are normally used to fulfil two main purposes:

1. *To establish the identity of the cardholder* (e.g. name, photograph, etc.). A unique identifier used on most debit and credit cards is the primary account number (PAN). It is usually a 16-digit number embossed on the front of the plastic card, and it is also stored (unencrypted) on the magnetic stripe of swipecards. The PAN is not a randomly generated number; it has to satisfy a mathematical formula known as the 'Luhn algorithm', essentially a check

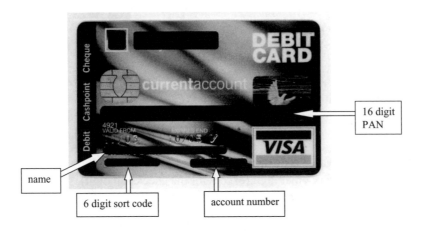

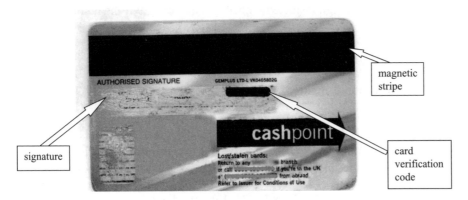

Figure 7.4 Key features of a debit card

on the last digit of the PAN. The reverse is not necessarily true: just because a number satisfies the algorithm does not mean that it will be accepted as a genuine PAN (despite the large number of 'credit card number generator' programs available through the internet). The first six (sometimes eight) digits contain information concerning the card issuer. For example, the first digit reflects the type of card issuer: if your debit card starts with a '4' or a '6' it probably means that it has been issued by a bank or similar financial institution. The remaining nine or so digits are unique to the cardholder, together with the final digit as a checksum for the Luhn algorithm.

Example of the Luhn Algorithm for a 16 digit PAN

Robin Bryant

Suppose a credit card has a PAN number of:

4 1 2 3   8 5 6 7   1 9 1 0   1 3 1 2

The checksum value is the final number, ie '2' for this PAN.
Next, double every other digit (except for the checksum digit), starting with the first digit. This gives:

8 1 4 3   16 5 12 7   2 9 2 0   2 3 2 2

Next, make each digit a single number by subtracting 9 if the number is 10 or bigger:

8 1 4 3   7 5 3 7   2 9 2 0   2 3 2 2

Now add all these digits together: $8+1+4+3+7+5+3+7+2+9+2+0+2+3+2+2 = \mathbf{60}$

If this number is divisible by 10 with no remainder then this could be a valid credit card number. As 60/10 is exactly 6 then this **could** be a valid number.
However, if the final number is changed to '3' the PAN becomes

4 1 2 3   8 5 6 7   1 9 1 0   1 3 1 3

This cannot be a valid credit card number as the sum would be 61, which is not divisible by 10.

2. *To check the cardholder's knowledge of the account* (signature, passwords, mother's maiden name etc.). The four digit Personal Identification Number (PIN) is a common means of checking account knowledge, and for obvious reasons, the PIN is not usually found on the magnetic stripe of swipe cards, although some card issuers do include information on parts of the magnetic stripe as a mathematical check on the PIN (an 'offset' value). However security protected information relating to the PIN, in non plaintext form, may be stored within the chip on a chip and PIN card.

Some parts of the plastic card industry refer to these two checks when combined as the CVM (customer verification method). The card often fulfils a third purpose:

3. *Authorisation.* There are a number of ways that this may be checked using a card, particularly for higher value transactions. A typical checking procedure (Visa, 2003) is shown in figure 7.5.

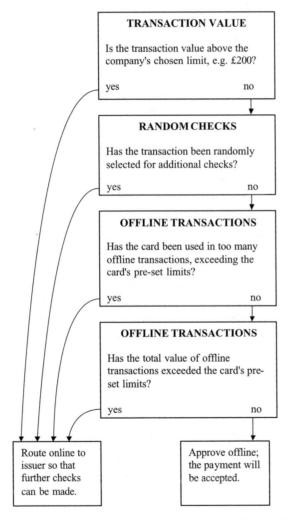

Figure 7.5   Point of sale checks for transactions using credit and debit cards

Chip and PIN

Chip and PIN cards incorporate a chip containing information linked to the customer's PIN and identity, and card issuer details. The four digit PIN must be entered each time the card is used at a 'point of sale' (POS) or at an ATM. The method used for verification of a chip and PIN transaction depends on the level of security required or when certain criteria are met. The PIN may be checked against either an encrypted version of the PIN stored within the chip, or checked against details stored by the card issuer, or possibly both.

Because it is not always considered necessary to check the PIN electronically with the issuer, the PIN is instead checked using the algorithms of the smart card and reader; the checking process can be quick, indicated by a rapid 'PIN OK' message to the user. This message has been removed from many pin-pads, presumably for reasons of security (to avoid drawing attention to the fact that the PIN is stored on the chip in some form), although it can still sometimes be observed when making small value purchases or when a card is used abroad.

When a higher level of security is required, the transaction process will take longer; a customer may have to wait a while after placing the card in a terminal and entering the PIN. If required, an encrypted PAN and/or PIN (a 'cryptogram') can be checked online with the issuing organisation by in effect sending an email. The circumstances when this is likely to happen are set out within the 'Visa EU Smart Payment Product Principles' (Visa, 2003), see figure 7.5. Most UK banks use static data authentication (SDA) chip and PIN cards which send the PIN to the card in plaintext form after entry at the keypad (Murdoch, 2007). More secure (but more expensive) smart cards use dynamic data authentication (DDA) or combined data authentication (CDA), which will encrypt the PIN.

To help prevent crimes involving the use of copied card details (most particularly, card not present (CNP) crimes), an additional three (occasionally four) digit card verification value (CVV) or card verification code (CVC) number is now printed on the back of credit and debit cards, often referred to as the 'three-digit security code' or the 'verification number'. It is usually found in the same section of the card that contains the signature, immediately after a repeat of the final four digits of the PAN, and is often requested when making online purchases.

7.2 Card crime

Crime involving plastic cards has probably been in existence since the inception of the cards themselves. As we note elsewhere in this book, technological change is often accompanied by criminal entrepreneurship. An early and crude type of plastic card fraud involved mechanically transferring the embossed details of the PAN from one card to another, a technique which became known colloquially as 'shave and paste'. Even simpler was the practice of stealing a card whilst it was in transit between a bank and the customer; banks soon introduced a system where the initial PIN was sent separately from the card itself. None of these early criminal techniques exploited the digital nature of credit cards. However, by the mid 1990s new techniques began to be developed, techniques that enabled fraudsters and others to access and reproduce the electronic information stored on some plastic cards. A 'skimmer' (see below) can be used to capture card data, providing the basis for creating cloned cards or committing other forms of fraud. Today skimmers are widely available through the internet; a search on the online US eBay auction house in September 2007 provided at least nine offers of hand-held 'credit card encoders' for sale.

Estimates vary on the current cost of plastic card crime in the UK but all agree that it is significant. For example, the association APACS estimated that card fraud losses in the UK amounted to £423 million (APACS, 2007b).

In this section, we will examine two forms of plastic card crime that have been particularly affected by changes in technology: swipe card and smart card crime.

7.2.1 Swipe card crime

Before the advent of more recent smart card technology, most conventional forms of swipe card fraud consisted of stealing the card and then making purchases assuming the identity of the owner. This relies on the fact that comparing signatures is a particularly imprecise check on identity; signatures change and develop, and POS staff are often unwilling to challenge a signature that differs from the version on the back of the card. (Readers who travel abroad may have noticed that in some countries POS staff rarely make any attempt to check the signature at all.)

If the fraudster knows the PIN, perhaps by shoulder-surfing prior to stealing the card (or on occasions exploiting the fact that the PIN may have been written on the card by the user) then the card can be used to make ATM withdrawals.

These types of fraud are often short lived as they involve stealing the plastic card, usually noticed by the victim within a short period of time, who subsequently reports the loss to the card issuer for cancellation.

Skimming

In the mid to late 1990s, when the technology became widely available (facilitated by the distribution of information over the internet), new forms of swipe card crime developed. Skimming involves copying the details of a credit card stored on the magnetic stripe by swiping the card through an electronic reader. Once the details (the PAN, the expiry date (if available) and the PIN (rarely if ever available from the stripe)) have been obtained, fraudsters may then create a duplicate card for their own use, particularly for 'card not present' transactions, conducted over the telephone or internet. The original card owner is unaware that the card has been skimmed and copied and so will not cancel the card, providing a window of opportunity for the fraudster. Unless the victim checks their account on-line or at an ATM, the first time a victim is likely to realise anything untoward has occurred is on receipt of a statement, which may be weeks later.

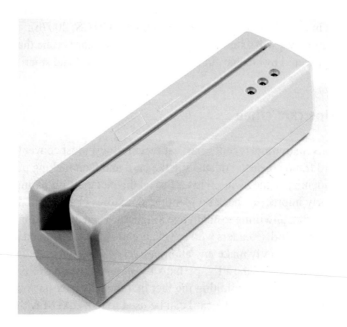

Figure 7.6   A handheld skimmer

Skimming can be carried out in two main ways, using either a dedicated hand-held device (a skimmer) or a genuine card reader connected to a storage device. Two historically popular circumstances for skimming are ATM skimmers and in-person service industry skimmers.

ATM skimmers are discreet devices placed over the card slot of an ATM so that the customer's card details are scanned and stored by the illegal hardware before (or after) the card enters the bank's card reader. The scanner may even be accompanied by a small camera to record the PIN entered by the victim. In 2005, four members of an ATM card skimming group were jailed for four years, having committed £200 000 worth of fraud (Leydon, 2005).

This type of fraud has been well publicised and warnings are placed on and near some ATMs asking customers not to use the machine if it looks in any way unusual. If there are signs of an ATM skimmer, the police advise the public to take no action apart from reporting it to the authorities; a skimmer is a valuable device and the criminal owner may intervene and become violent if a person were to attempt to remove or damage the equipment. Because of their value, there is also a very good chance that the crook will return to retrieve the machine (even if the stolen data has been transmitted wirelessly); the police may then have a chance to arrest the fraudster.

Most in-person service industry skimmers have been reported as working in petrol stations and restaurants (BBC, 2000a, 2000b). A particularly popular method involves taking the card away when offered in payment for a restaurant meal; the card is skimmed (and used in a genuine transaction), and then returned to the user. Even if the card is not taken away, it may still be skimmed; the skimmer may be not much bigger than a credit card, and can be discreetly attached in line with the genuine card reader. Alternatively, a genuine card reader may be attached to a data storage device; as the card is swiped to make a payment, the PAN is transmitted and stored for later use by the fraudster.

The advantage the CVC code is that in order to quote the code you usually have to be in possession of the card itself; the code is not stored on the magnetic stripe and hence it is not available through electronic skimming. (However, it is obvious that CVC may be simply noted by the fraudster if the card is handed over for out of sight processing, and then either written down or stored in a key pad).

Another common method of obtaining card details, supposedly used until relatively recently and often reported in the media, involves collecting plastic card details from discarded receipts, bank statements and other documents. A practice referred to in north America as 'dumpster diving' is (or was) apparently used to collect this information (dumpster is the American term for a rubbish skip). Despite the fact that there have been few independent accounts of the phenomenon,

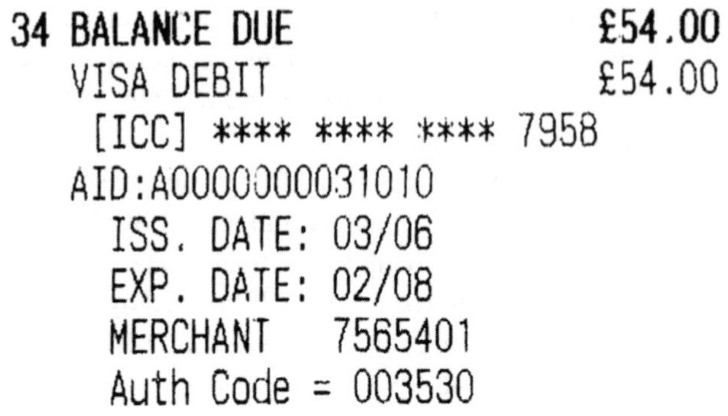

```
34 BALANCE DUE                          £54.00
   VISA DEBIT                           £54.00
   [ICC] **** **** **** 7958
 AID:A0000000031010
   ISS. DATE: 03/06
   EXP. DATE: 02/08
   MERCHANT   7565401
   Auth Code = 003530
```

Figure 7.7   Extract from a shop receipt

the full PAN is no longer printed on receipts; the majority of the numerals are replaced by asterisks instead, leaving (typically) just the last four digits for any subsequent query by the customer, see figure 7.8 as an example.

7.2.2 Smart card crime

Smart cards have been the target of a number of criminal practices, particularly in the late 1990s with the manufacture of illegal cloned and 'everlasting' phonecards. More recently, chip and PIN credit and debit cards have been the target of fraudsters.

An early example of smart card crime was to gain unauthorised access to pay-TV services, particularly those offered by British Sky Broadcasting (BSkyB or 'Sky TV') before the advent of digital services. In the mid 1990s, BSkyB employed the videocrypt system for encrypting (or 'scrambling') their services. Although the association between a particular receiver and the chip on the smart card (see above) provides a relatively robust system, it can be compromised with sufficient knowledge of the architecture of the systems employed and the mathematical algorithms used for encryption and decryption. The company appeared at the outset to have full confidence in their videocrypt system; however in early 1993 key information concerning the encryption (the hash functions) was somehow released into the public domain (see Kuhn, 1996). This information allowed a PC-based emulation of genuine Sky TV cards, using a hardware interface linking the card reader in the satellite receiver to a serial port of the computer, and then running a relatively simple program.

The flat end of the interface (on the right) is inserted into the smart card reader; the eight contact connectors can be seen. (They are read from the underside, so

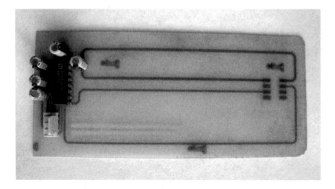

Figure 7.8 A smart card reader interface

the configuration of the connectors shown on this interface is the mirror image of the configuration shown in figure 7.3; on the interface shown here, C1 is at the top right and C5 is at the top left).

In effect the PC would perform the calculations usually undertaken by a Sky TV conditional access card, 'fooling' the videocrypt CAM into assuming that it was communicating with a genuine card. The decrypting programs were known at the time as 'Season' software. This was allegedly an oblique reference to attempts by non-UK European viewers to view the Star Trek 'Season' TV series. (Sky TV, who enjoyed exclusive rights to the Star Trek series, do not allow viewers outside the UK and Ireland to subscribe to their services.) However, given the nature of the 'homebrew' equipment involved and the necessity to have at least some rudimentary knowledge of running software, this particular approach to hacking remained largely at the 'amateur' or enthusiast level.

However, demand for Sky TV services from non-UK residents (particularly British expatriates living in Spain) remained at a high level, despite the official line that access cards could not be sold to those living outside of the UK or Ireland. This demand was met, at least in part, by the supply of standalone (pirate) devices which effectively contained a programmable microchip (often a Motorola PIC) able to provide the correct responses to the videocrypt data requests, and obviated the need for a PC to be connected. These devices steadily became more sophisticated, smaller and more 'user-friendly' in terms of any code updates necessary (after Sky TV began electronic counter measures, ECMs). Eventually they became programmable smart cards with an embedded chip, often known as 'gold' cards, only distinguishable from the 'real thing' by the lack of a company logo and other identifying features. Other similar 'wafer' cards (available in a range of colours) were used to make fraudulent payments, such as video rental payments.

Figure 7.9   A 'Gold card'

Whereas the earlier PC-based approaches to hacking the Sky TV system were largely conducted by hobbyist or 'amateur' communities and had little illegal application, pirate access cards were a different matter. They were of obvious interest to those wishing to supply access to Sky TV services to customers who were either prevented from obtaining a legal subscription (living in other parts of Europe) or who wished to gain free and illegal access to the paid TV programmes. Some cards also 'opened up' the full range of subscription services utilising the same videocrypt encryption system, (beyond those of Sky TV) such as the Japanese TV channel JSTV.

In 1998, Harold (Chris) Cary, described by a judge as a leading manufacturer and vendor of pirate smart cards in the mid 1990s, was jailed for 4 years after being found guilty of conspiracy to defraud BSkyB of £30 million (Irish Independent, 1998). However, the relationship (if any) between hobbyists who helped to uncover the details of the videocrypt encryption processes, and subsequent more organised activities of those (such as Cary) who sourced and supplied pirate cards, was far from clear. At the turn of the last century, the now defunct terrestrial digital TV service 'ITV Digital' became the victim of widespread piracy of its conditional access smart cards (McAuliffe, 2001).

Although the current system used by Sky TV (which has moved entirely to digital TV standards and now employs the Videoguard system) appears to have withstood any attempts to circumvent its conditional access systems, other Pay TV systems have not proved so robust. For example, in Italy in 2002 it was estimated that 4.1 million households viewed Pay TV but only 1.9 million were legally subscribing (Italmedia Consulting, cited by Loebbecke and Fischer,

2005). The industry pressure group, the Association Européenne pour la Protection des Œuvres et services Cryptés (AEPOC) estimates that approximately 1 billion Euros are spent each year on pirate cards and devices for unlocking Pay TV services in Europe (AEPOC, 2007a). AEPOC also claims that there are 'thousands of European websites ... pertaining to piracy of audiovisual services and offer software, access codes, tips and tricks and other relevant information to the hackers' (AEPOC, 2007b). In 2004 piracy in the US was estimated to be costing the DirecTV provider $1.2 billion per year in lost revenues (Poulson, 2004). The digitalisation of satellite TV services (leading to a much greater number of channels and market penetration) is correlated with an increase in piracy. Concerns have also been expressed that because of shared digital technologies (amongst other reasons) TV piracy might 'spread' from satellite TV to other digital TV platforms, such as terrestrial and cable forms of distribution (European Commission, 2003).

In 2007 a clearer distinction may be made between:

- 'professional pirates' who employ sophisticated methods and equipment to produce pirate cards on a commercial scale;

- 'local manufacturers' who produce 'DIY' pirate cards and who are heavily dependent on the internet for information;

- 'home industry pirates' who see cracking the Pay TV coding systems as an intellectual challenge, and who are also active on internet forums (Loebbecke and Fischer, 2005).

Nonetheless, it has been suggested that a form of symbiotic relationship exists between the professional pirates and local manufacturers; the latter being used as a means of distribution of illegal cards (European Commission, 2003).

Chip and PIN card crime

According to the Association of Payment Clearing Services (APACS, 2006), the introduction of chip and PIN reduced losses through cloned, stolen and lost cards by 24%, or £58.4 million. There have been no recorded instances of cloning chips, but chip and PIN cards with a magnetic stripe are not immune to ATM fraud, (Leydon, 2006). Any chip and PIN credit or debit card with a magnetic stripe can be skimmed, and the copied details be used to make a duplicate card for ATM withdrawals abroad. This is possible because many ATMs outside the

UK have not been updated to recognise an embedded microchip and rely instead on the magnetic stripe. Card owners may be under the impression that a card with a chip is inherently more secure, but this is clearly not always the case; a combination swipe and smart card is as vulnerable to skimming and copying as a simple swipe card, as in some cases the sophisticated security available through the chip is just ignored.

In addition, new methods have been developed for gaining knowledge of the PIN. At a POS or ATM, the PIN is entered by the customer in plain text form, and the PIN may then be encrypted (but often is not) and transmitted to the card issuer for checking (see above). However, before the PIN is encrypted, and especially if it is not, there is an obvious danger of intercepting the plaintext traffic within the pad itself. Manufacturers are aware of this, and the pads are designed to be tamper proof; however Shell suspended its chip and PIN payments in 2006 as 1 million pounds of customers' money had gone missing (BBC, 2006). The BBC also reported that the Sri Lankan Tamil Tigers may be responsible for a card cloning scam (BBC, 2007). Although the precise details of the hack remain unclear, researchers at Cambridge University seem to have shown that hacking of chip and PIN pinpads is at least theoretically possible (Bond, 2006; Drimer, 2006).

There are less technologically dependent ways in which chip and PIN smart card crime may be perpetrated. For example, simply shoulder-surfing the PIN, stealing the card and then using the card and PIN to make cash withdrawals and purchases is still possible. And in many ways, crime enacted with a chip and PIN card is potentially more damaging to an individual than earlier swipe card crime. This is because in the past a PIN was effectively only used at an ATM, but now it is used much more widely. Shoulder-surfing for the PIN is being counteracted by making both retailers and users more aware of the danger (e.g. APACS, 2007a) and increasing privacy around the pinpad.

Chip and PIN initiatives have inevitably had little effect on CNP fraud, for the obvious reason that these transactions (often by phone or online) do not involve reading the chip, and instead rely upon the PAN and CVC for customer identity verification. According to the industry body APACS, CNP fraud now represents the largest form of credit fraud in the UK (APACS, 2007b).

7.3 Investigating card crime

It is widely acknowledged in the UK that the police are unable to investigate all reported plastic credit and debit card offences (e.g. City of London Police, 2005). In effect, these crimes are 'screened' and a decision made concerning whether to conduct further investigations. For obvious reasons the exact criteria used for screening are not normally in the public domain. Apart from the obvious criteria relating to seriousness and frequency, a police force policy is also likely to be mindful of the National Intelligence Model (NIM) for policing. Under the NIM, crimes are categorised according to Level 1 (crimes that affect a single division or area of a police force), Level 2 (crimes at the force or regional level) or Level 3 (crimes of a national or international level).

Level 1 and Level 2 plastic card crimes, if investigated, are likely to be tackled by a force-based unit, variously called a 'Fraud Squad', an 'Economic Crime Unit' or a 'Cheque and Plastic Card Fraud Team' and the like. Any Level 3 plastic card related crime is likely to be passed to the Serious Organised Crime Agency (SOCA) for investigation. There has recently been some suggestion (and even criticism) that in future, screening for further investigation might be carried out by the banks and other financial institutions themselves, rather than by the police (Caulfield, 2007). The industry itself already supplements the police resources available to investigate plastic card crime. For example, the industry body APACS sponsors the work of the Dedicated Cheque and Plastic Crime Unit (DCPCU)

Although there are examples of a number of high profile criminal prosecutions of individuals illegally selling cards to access Pay TV it would appear that most of the initiative in combating this type of crime has been taken by the companies themselves. This normally includes using ECMs or introducing new versions of CAMs and the associated software. For example, the Viaccess encryption system (used by a number of European satellite TV providers) is currently at version 4, the previous three versions having been compromised in a variety of ways. There are however, examples of more proactive action by satellite TV providers to protect their services. Chris Cary absconded from open prison, but was subsequently recaptured in New Zealand by private investigators hired by BSkyB and returned to the UK to serve the rest of his sentence (Benetto, 1999). In the US cable TV viewers using pirate cards received an onscreen message to phone a toll-free 800 number (no charge) to receive a free tee-shirt whereas official subscribers did not (a 'silver bullet' approach). Those responding to the on screen message inadvertently supplied their details to the company concerned (Anderson, 2001, p. 428).

Questions

Robin Bryant & Sarah Bryant

1. What is the 'fallback' fraud?

2. In fraud terms, why do customers prefer signatures but the banks prefer the PIN? Do you accept the banks' argument?

3. Explain (in everyday terms) why SDA is an inherently weaker approach to bank card security than DDA. Which system do most UK banks apparently use?

4. Why is 'shoulder-surfing' (including the consequences) a potentially bigger problem with chip and PIN than with previous card payment methods?

5. What are two examples in the UK of 'CNP' fraud?

6. When a payment is refused off line, how does the system 'know' what purchases have been made earlier in the day?

7. What is a 'gold card'?

References

AEPOC (2007a) The Problem of Piracy Against Conditional Access Systems. [Online]. Available at: http://www.aepoc.org/index2.htm (Accessed: Oct 10 2007).

AEPOC (2007b) Press Backgrounder Piracy, Pay-TV and AEPOC.[Online]. Available at: http://www.aepoc.org/index2.htm (Accessed: Oct 10 2007).

Anderson, R. (2001) *Security Engineering: A Guide to Building Dependable Distributed Systems.* New York: John Wiley & Sons.

APACS (2006) Press Releases – UK card fraud losses in 2005 fall by £65m. [Online]. Available at: http://www.apacs.org.uk/media_centre/press/06_03_07.html (Accessed: Aug 3 2007).

APACS (2007a) Transactions with your chip and PIN terminal. [Online]. Available at: http://www.apacs.org.uk/documents/RetailerPOSadviceguide.pdf (Accessed: Oct 10 2007).

APACS (2007b) Card Fraud Facts and Figures. [Online]. Available at: http://www.apacs.org.uk/resources_publications/card_fraud_facts_and_figures.html (Accessed: Oct 10 2007).

BBC (2000a) Computer chips 'fight card con waiters'. BBC News [Online]. Available at: http://news.bbc.co.uk/1/hi/uk/809900.stm (Accessed: Aug 3 2007).

BBC (2000b) Card fraud problems expected to escalate before Christmas. BBC News [Online]. Available at: http://www.bbc.co.uk/devon/news/122000/19/fraud.shtml (Accessed: Aug 3 2007).

BBC (2006) Petrol firm suspends chip-and-pin. BBC News [Online]. Available at: http://news.bbc.co.uk/1/hi/england/4980190.stm (Accessed: Aug 3 2007).

BBC (2007) Motorists hit by card clone scam. BBC News [Online]. Available at: http://news.bbc.co.uk/1/hi/uk/6578595.stm (Accessed: Aug 3 2007).

Benetto, J. (1999) BSkyB cheat is dished by Murdoch. [Online]. Available at: http://findarticles.com/p/articles/mi_qn4158/is_19990109/ai_n9656534 (Accessed: Oct 10 2007).

Bond, M. (2006) Chip and PIN (EMV) point-of-sale terminal interceptor. [Online]. Available at: http://www.cl.cam.ac.uk/~mkb23/interceptor/ (Accessed: Oct 10 2007).

Caulfield, P. (2007) Home Office accused of not investigating credit card fraud.[Online]. Available at: http://www.24dash.com/billpayments/22639.htm (Accessed: Oct 10 2007).

City of London Police (2005) Cheque and credit card fraud investigation policy. [Online]. Available at: http://www.cityoflondon.police.uk/NR/rdonlyres/3528E395-EDE9–4B8C-A8BA-829C00982E0D/0/chequecreditcardfraudinvestigationFOI.pdf (Accessed: Oct 10 2007).

Drimer, S. (2006) Chip & PIN terminal playing Tetris. [Online]. Available at: http://www.lightbluetouchpaper.org/2006/12/24/chip-pin-terminal-playing-tetris (Accessed: Aug 3 2007).

European Commission (2003) On the legal protection of electronic pay services. Report from the Commission to the Council, the European Parliament and the European Economic and Social Committee [Online]. Available at: http://ec.europa.eu/internal_market/media/docs/elecpay/com-2003–198_en.pdf (Accessed: Oct 10 2007).

Irish Independent (1998) Ex-pirate radio chief jailed for £30m Sky card scam, April 3. [Online]. Available at: http://www.independent.ie/national-news/expirate-radio-chief-jailed-for-pound30m-sky-card-scam-447370.html (Accessed: Oct 10 2007).

Kuhn, M. (1996) Some technical details about Videocrypt. [Online]. Available at: http://www.cl.cam.ac.uk/~mgk25/tv-crypt/details.txt (Accessed: Oct 10 2007).

Leydon, J. (2005) £200K card skimming gang caged. [Online]. Available at: http://www.theregister.co.uk/2005/08/12/atm_scam_gang_jailed/ (Accessed: Aug 3 2007).

Leydon, J. (2006) Chip and PIN fraud hits Lloyds TSB. [Online]. Available at: http://www.theregister.co.uk/2006/05/11/lloyds_tsb_chip_and_pin_fraud/ (Accessed: Aug 3 2007).

Loebbecke, C. and Fischer, M. (2005) Business opportunities and risks from pay-TV piracy: the case of Europe. *Proceedings of the Eleventh Americas Conference on Information Systems,* Omaha, NE, USA August 11–14 2005.

McAuliffe, W. (2001) ITV Digital falls prey to smartcard piracy. [Online]. Available at: http://news.zdnet.co.uk/security/0,1000000189,2095655,00.htm (Accessed: Oct 10 2007).

Murdoch, S. (2007) EMV flaws and fixes: vulnerabilities in smart card payment systems. [Online]. Available at: http://www.cl.cam.ac.uk/~sjm217/talks/leuven07emv.pdf (Accessed: Oct 10 2007).

Poulson, K. (2004) DirecTV hacker sentenced to seven years. [Online]. Available at: http://www.securityfocus.com/news/10103 (Accessed: Oct 10 2007).

Visa (2003) Visa EU Smart Payment Product Principles Version 3.0 July 2003. [Online]. Available at: http://www.chipandpin.co.uk/reflib/SP3_main_brochure.pdf (Accessed: Oct 10 2007).

8

Telecommunications Fraud

Joe Carthy, Tahar Kechadi and Paul Gillen

Telecommunications fraud has become a crucial issue for investigators in recent years, computer crime investigation units across the world are increasingly inundated with reports of various types of telecommunications fraud. That is not to say that telecommunications fraud is a new phenomenon, but rather that both the telecommunications industry and the business community have recently seen fit to report incidents which hitherto went unreported; up until now such fraudulent activity, and the resulting loss of income or profit, has been absorbed and discreetly written off by the corporate sector. The European law enforcement community have struggled to investigate these frauds, given the limited availability of evidence, as well as limited formal training and tools.

The telecommunications industry has grown significantly over the past 20 years. This growth is based on the widespread deployment of technology, such as mobile devices, high-bandwidth fibre and intelligent private automatic branch exchange (PABX) systems, capable of delivering high-quality services to end-users. The trend continues with the development of voice and fax over internet protocol (VoIP/FoIP), 3G mobile technology and infrastructural developments such as Universal Mobile Telecommunications System (UMTS) and Internet Protocol version 6 (IPv6).

Inevitably, increasing levels of fraud have accompanied these advances, as criminals are attracted by the high value of communications services. With the proliferation of the internet and telecommunications systems, the breaching of

Investigating Digital Crime   Edited by Robin Bryant and Sarah Bryant
© 2008 John Wiley & Sons, Ltd

national borders by criminals has increased. Proper investigation by law enforcement agencies has been seriously hampered as national borders limit investigative powers and jurisdiction for each agency and nation. As a result of the growing trend in trans-national cybercrime, further legislative improvements will have to be made in order to assist investigations, particularly in areas such as the transfer of evidence and its admissibility across different jurisdictions.

The losses incurred by medium-sized companies have in some cases run to hundreds of thousands of euro per month. The profits for criminals are large and the risk of capture is small. In order to cope with this problem, the law enforcement community will probably need to develop new tools and procedures to investigate these frauds and tackle the organised criminals involved. This is essential to maintaining confidence in the global telecommunications system and can only be achieved by ensuring that systems are in place to deal with the problems.

Clearly the emerging information technology and telecommunications convergence provides many new opportunities for fraud. There is an ongoing need for research and development into methodologies and tools for the detection and investigation of these types of crime. One important category of telecommunications crime causing major corporate losses is PABX and/or voicemail fraud. Therefore particular methodologies to deal with this category of fraud are required; indeed such procedures might possibly provide a firm basis on which to develop suitable approaches for tackling other related types of fraud in the converged environment.

It is with that in mind we will examine:

- the methods used in the investigation of PABX fraud;

- the various methods used in the execution of the fraud; and

- the issues in relation to establishing effective approaches to the detection of this type of fraud.

8.1 Telecommunication systems and services

This section outlines how the telecommunications industry operates as well as examining some of the emerging technologies and current international developments.

8.1.1 Associated services

These are services that operate in conjunction with a telecommunications infrastructure, and include premium rate services and international simple voice
resellers.

Premium rate service

Premium rate service (PRS) is provided by companies or individuals on premium
rate telephone numbers. These special services include weather forecasting, traffic
news, stock exchange reports, sports results, live services (including services
of an adult nature), Tarot services, competition services, dating services and
messaging services. The total amount charged to the calling customer is shared
between:

- the carrier(s) of the call;

- the PRS service provider (i.e. the company who provide the PRS number(s) to
  the business client); and

- the business client to recover the costs of the service or services the business is
  providing.

This process is known as 'revenue share', and presents opportunities for fraud.

In the UK, the PRS numbers are (090X XXX) and these numbers are issued
or allocated by Oftel (Office of the Telecommunications Regulator) in blocks
of 1000. The numbers are then sub-allocated to service providers who in turn
may sell them onto business customers. This makes identification of active PRS
numbers difficult to establish (Telecommunications UK Fraud Forum Training
CD Version 1, 2001). In the UK, the Independent Committee for the Supervision
of Standards of Telephone Information Services (ICSTIS) supervises the
promotion and content of PRS on behalf of the telephone companies.

Fixed line, mobile, internet and SMS users can access premium rate services,
and the payment flow principle is the same in all cases. The cost of the call is
negotiable between the service provider and the operator up to a maximum set
by the regulatory authority in the particular jurisdiction.

International simple voice resellers

International services may be provided by an operator to customers using international network facilities owned by other operators. Such a provider is called an international simple voice reseller (ISVR). In the case of an outgoing call, the ISVR collects traffic from the public telecommunications operator (PTO), transfers it to a line leased from a facilities operator, and then hands it over to a PTO in an overseas country who will deliver the call to its destination. ISVR therefore involves breakout onto the public telecommunications network at both ends, but with the international leg of the call being carried on leased circuits. ISVR traffic bypasses the accounting rate system used for national calls.

8.1.2 Interconnect and payment flows

It is not practical for every service provider to own dedicated lines to each country in the world. Therefore a system of interconnection between service providers and payment flows had to be established to ensure streamlining of services and international connectivity.

In simple terms the telecommunications service providers make use of other providers' infrastructures and pay 'interconnect charges' for this facility. On a national basis this principle is used when subscribers opt for a 'preferred carrier' other than the national carrier (or the carrier that actually owns the infrastructure, for example BT in the UK). A preferred carrier is simply a telecommunications carrier of choice.

Telecommunications companies use the existing network connectivity to deliver their services to areas in which they do not themselves have the infrastructure to connect directly within their own network. In this way, telecommunication service providers are able to connect to and to transit calls to and from other providers' customers.

This practice allows for wider connectivity than if each telecommunications operator was required to provide the necessary infrastructure to perform sole connectivity between every point worldwide. The principle of interconnection is to successfully complete the connection and routing of a call from one customer to another, regardless of the telecommunications networks used by these customers. The negotiation of interconnect agreements and costs is a commercial responsibility, with each telecommunications operator usually having a department or number of people assigned to this task.

Interconnectivity is a key issue in telecommunications fraud; the connectivity between service providers is an Achilles' heel in the investigation of telecommunications fraud. This issue will be discussed later but it is important to bear it in mind as a cornerstone in the operation of the telecommunication system.

Figure 8.1 shows a typical scenario where a telecommunications carrier does not have a dedicated network over which it owns all the connectivity. (All charges are notional and the scenario does not represent real agreements among the mentioned providers.) In this scenario Eircom in Ireland wants to offer calling to Algeria to its customers and also wants to be able to transit calls to Algeria for other operators. Eircom has no direct connectivity in place to do this, and to provide direct connectivity would increase the cost of terminating calls to Algeria to its customers.

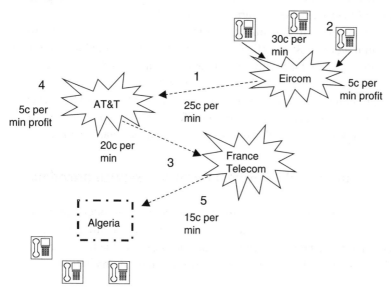

Figure 8.1 Interconnectivity between service providers

The system operates as follows:

- Eircom, who have an established business relationship with AT&T in North America, are aware that their preferred carrier is offering favourable rates to Algeria at 25c per minute (rates for demonstration purposes only). These rates are covered in the appropriate interconnect agreement. Eircom can now offer calls to Algeria to its customers for say 30c per minute, making 5c per minute on each call after paying AT&T 25c per minute.

- AT&T, who have no direct links to Algeria, are able to transit calls through France Télécom in France, their 'preferred carrier', at favourable rates of 20c per minute. These rates are the subject of the Interconnect Agreement between AT&T and France Télécom. AT&T are able to make 5c per minute after receiving 25c from Eircom and paying France Télécom 20c.

- France Télécom is able to terminate the calls directly to Algeria because they have direct connectivity and this costs them 15c per minute. Therefore as a result of the various agreements and costs, France Télécom is able to make 5c per minute.

In this way, Eircom customers experience a seamless service to Algeria and are unaware of the routes used to terminate their calls.

Each company will sell minutes to the previous operator at slightly higher rates than it would cost to deliver to the next operator or final terminating point. All negotiations are done within the interconnect agreements and settlements are made for the costs of the calls between each operator. The practice of buying and selling call minutes is known as 're-filing'. In this context, 'preferred carriers' are carriers that telecoms operators would prefer to use due to the rates offered, the quality of service and established favourable business relationships.

8.1.3 Regulation of telecommunications service providers

In every jurisdiction the telecommunication service providers are regulated by statutory agencies and self-regulation. In the UK the regulators are Oftel and ICSTIS, described below. Similar organisations exist in the rest of Europe, under the EU's regulatory framework for the telecommunications industry.

Oftel

The Office of Telecommunications (Oftel) is the regulator for the UK telecommunications industry, and operates under the UK Telecommunications Act 1984. Its duties and responsibilities include:

- developing policies on telecommunications;

- ensuring telecommunications service providers meet their obligations under telecommunications and competition laws and regulations;

- promoting the interest of users;

- maintaining and promoting effective competition;

- ensuring that telecommunications services are provided to meet all 'reasonable demands' including access to emergency services, provision of public call boxes and services in rural areas and providing directory information.

Oftel hold all licence records needed by telecommunications service providers issued by the Department of Trade and Industry in the UK.

ICSTIS

ICSTIS is the Independent Committee for the Supervision of Standards of Telephone Information Services and is the industry-funded regulatory body for all premium rate charged telecommunications services in the UK. It is a non-profit-making body and consists of part-time committee members, supported by a full time secretariat.

ICSTIS regulates the content and promotion of services through a Code of Practice. Its roles include investigating complaints and it has the power to fine companies and bar access to services.

8.2 Telecommunications crime

There are a variety of crimes that have been perpetrated against every available telephone service over the years. A brief description of the crimes and some examples are given below. PABX fraud is described in more detail.

- *Long distance telephone fraud via the internet* is a relatively recent type of telecommunications fraud. Typically, the injured party downloads a program from the internet which claims to have site-specific features. The program installs itself after the user clicks past a disclaimer. (It is also possible that downloading can occur without the knowledge of the injured party.) Once the program is installed it hijacks the modem and disconnects from the user's normal service provider and reconnects via an alternative service provider. The alternative service provider will typically be in an international location; calls will be to a premium rate service and will be charged at that premium rate. This type of fraud will impact on users who have a dial up connection to the internet. An example of such a fraud and its investigation is provided in section 4.1, and further details are available in Ó Ciardhuáin and Gillen (2002).

- *Prepaid calling card fraud* is perpetrated against individuals who have bought such cards to make reduced rate prepaid international calls. The call cards themselves are not needed to make the call; only the username and PIN are needed. Thieves steal the call card PIN by hanging around hotel lobbies, airport call kiosks, rail kiosks or other public telephones. Fraudsters have been known to use binoculars to see numbers being entered in public phones. The prepaid balance on the call card can then be used to make international calls.

- *Clip-on fraud* is the rerouting of lines using alligator clips, from a call kiosk or a telephone junction box to another location, such as a call selling operation offering cheap international calls to immigrants calling home. The simplest type of clip on fraud occurred in call kiosks; fraudsters clipped on to the line in the kiosk and used their own handset to sell international calls to pre-arranged customers.

- *Subscription fraud* is a time-honoured scam where a customer signs up for service with no intention to pay for it. It is in itself a very large area but the techniques and issues involved in its investigation are largely outside the scope of this present work. Subscription fraud can vary from simple to complex. More complex scams include setting up fraudulent businesses, often with fake identification and fake credit references. Other scams include using real names and companies to obtain telephone services with the intention not to pay for service. In most cases, call sell operations will net a profit on the service in use during a 30-day period, following which the victim (on receipt of the telephone bill) becomes aware of the fraud (Telecommunications UK Fraud Forum Training CD Version 1, 2001). Generally these types of fraud can be investigated using conventional investigative procedures since the fraud itself is not dependent on the technology.

- *Mobile phone fraud* comes in many guises. The most common type of mobile phone fraud concerns the use of prepaid mobile phones where users obtain service by obtaining credit by the use of stolen or compromised credit cards. Other offences related to mobile phones are covered in Chapter 11.

- *Premium rate service fraud* can take a number of forms and the injured parties can be the subscribers or the telecommunications service providers.

Unsuspecting victims may be persuaded to call premium rate service numbers to claim fictitious prizes. Alternatively, a computer modem is diverted to call a PRS, as in the long distance telephone scam mentioned above.

- *Call forwarding scams* have been reported in the USA and may operate in several ways. For example, an impostor calls a customer attempting to persuade the customer to reveal the PIN on his or her call forward feature. Armed with this PIN, the impostor can forward the customer's telephone to various international destinations. International calls can then be made through the customer's phone. Another method of operating this scam is performed by the impostor leaving an automated message on the customer's voice mail system about claiming a prize. The message instructs the victim to dial a two-digit code followed by a hash or an asterisk, and then to dial a particular phone number. The number is the long distance operator and the two-digit code is the local service provider's code for call forwarding. The impostor will then dial the customer's number and be forwarded to the long distance operator; the scam artist can then make international calls at the customer's expense.

- *Slamming* is an American term for a type of telephone fraud that involves changing a subscriber's telephone service provider without permission. The *modus operandi* may involve a customer receiving a call from a telemarketer asking the customer to change long-distance telephone service provider. Although the subscriber is not interested in the change (and makes this clear to the telemarketer), the service provider is changed anyway.

- *Cramming* is an American term for a fraud committed by a telecommunications company. The company bills a customer for services not used or ordered. It is called cramming because the fraudulent charges are squeezed or crammed onto the bill along with other normal charges in an effort to get customers to overlook fees.

- *Boxing* scams usually entailed adding a 'box' to a system either electronically or physically to obtain free calls through the manipulation of the signalling system of the analogue telephone network. As noted in an earlier chapter, the most famous example was 'Blue Boxing'; and the most well known exponent a US phreaker using the name Cap'n Crunch (US Department of Defense, 1985).

  The Blue Box was so named because of the colour of the first one obtained by the authorities. Figure 8.2 shows one example of a 'blue' box made from a modified calculator. A typical blue box had 12 or 13 buttons or switches that

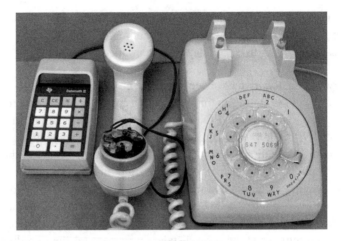

Figure 8.2 A 'blue box' (Courtesy of Bob McGarrah; reproduced with permission.)

emitted the tones used in the normal operation of the telephone long distance network at the time. This effectively allowed the user to become the operator of the phone line. The device could be directly connected to the phone line or alternatively acoustically connected to a telephone handset by placing the Blue Box speaker next to the transmitter or the telephone handset. The device would emulate the 2600 Hz signal used to clear the line establishing the on-hook or off-hook condition of the line. The operator of the device would then emit the various DTMF tones representing numbers, and then press the ST key to indicate that all the digits had been sent; the equipment would then start connecting to the called number. The advent of digital networks saw the demise of this early scam.

8.2.1 PABX fraud

PABX fraud is one of the more serious frauds to affect businesses. A company falling victim to PABX fraud can suffer severe financial loss. In Ireland, statistics from the Garda Computer Crime Investigation Unit (CCIU, unpublished) reveal that there has been an increase in PABX fraud; cases currently under investigation at the CCIU involve approximately €3.5 m in losses to the injured parties. This figure only takes into account those companies who have reported the offences; it is believed that unreported losses in Ireland run to between €6 and €10 million per annum. These estimated figures are based on intelligence from telecommunications carriers and information supplied by police services (the Gardaí working in conjunction with law enforcement agencies abroad). In many of these cases the injured parties may never have intended to report the attack to the Gardaí, but have been identified in the course of wider investigations.

It is not only private companies that are at risk; in Ireland the Gardaí are currently investigating complaints from government departments. The report of the Irish Comptroller and Auditor General for the year 2002 disclosed that the Department of Social and Family Affairs had been the victim of a toll fraud on their PABX system, and had accrued losses amounting to an estimated €294 136 (Comptroller and Auditor General, 2003).

The Metropolitan Police in London were hacked in a PABX fraud and this attack resulted in a loss of £1 million sterling. The culprits were never caught. As is generally the case, these attacks originated from abroad and have ceased before the injured party even becomes aware of it. Additional problems exist when it comes to tracing the source and deciding what offence, if any, has taken place.

PABX systems

A PABX is a sophisticated computer-based switchboard that can be thought of as a small in-house phone company for the organisation. PABX systems are widespread throughout government and business. Connected to the PSTN, the PABX provides organisation and routing of internal calls, the transfer of incoming calls to the destination extension and the forwarding of outgoing calls to their destination through the PSTN. Among other features it also allows an authorised user to access the internal network from outside and make telephone calls over the company's lines.

PABX vulnerabilities

Modern digital PABX systems, like computer systems, offer a host of capabilities, many of which the average user is unaware. These new features effectively offer new opportunities for an attacker to exploit (phreak) a PABX system, using the features for a purpose for which they were never intended (NIST, 1999, 2000). The threats to government and businesses using PABX systems include:

- *Theft of service*; toll fraud is probably the most common motive for attackers.

- *Traffic analysis*; passive monitoring of the traffic on the PABX may include gathering intelligence on a company.

- *Denial of service attacks*; any action that impairs the operation of the PABX, perhaps with a view to extortion.

- *Unauthorised access*; to system resources or privileges.

- *Data modification*; modification of system routing tables to gain additional services.

- *Disclosure of information*; eavesdropping on calls.

A successful PABX phreak enables the phreaker to route international telephone calls through a PABX system and out onto other telephone lines. These calls can then be sold on a minute-by-minute basis in a call shop, providing substantial profits to the seller. The company who own the targeted PABX system unwittingly incur the cost of these calls and substantial losses are likely to have been sustained before the hack comes to light. The culprit meanwhile simply moves on to the next target.

PABX features particularly exploited by phreakers include:

- DISAs or Dial In System Access lines; facilities which allow employees or maintenance contractors to access the telephone system externally. A user connects to the DISA port, inputs a pass code and is allocated an outgoing trunk telephone line which allows them to make outgoing calls over the company's network or enables essential maintenance to be carried out remotely, without having to be present at the company's premises.

- Voice mail, effectively the company answering machine. It consists of a small computer that records messages and relays messages to the destination extension in a telephone network, often requiring the input of a pass code. voice mail boxes (VMBs) are separate user accounts on a voice mail system including an administrator account, which allows for the creation of new accounts and the deletion of existing ones.

Phreaking a PABX

The most common method of entry to a PABX system is either through voice mail or DISA lines. In the case of voice mail, the abuser accesses an existing VMB using a PIN cracker and, providing administration settings allow, starts making calls. With DISA, the abuser simply has to access a DISA line by means of a wardialler (using a computer program to dial a large number of telephone numbers in a succession), and then check the system to confirm if access to a DISA line is granted. The hacker can then store successful attempts for future large-scale use.

Attacks on PABX systems are many and varied, but technical examinations reveal that in the majority of reported cases offenders dial into the PABX system from outside, create external lines and then make large numbers of outgoing international calls. Limited technical knowledge is required as the necessary methodological information is readily available from system manuals, and from dedicated hackers' sites and computer security sites on the internet. (The only difference in the information on these sites is the angle taken in the delivery of the information, i.e. the hackers' sites provide information on how to hack, while the computer security sites offer guidance on how to prevent attacks. Both types of site give enough information to attempt a hack.) Typical well-known hacker/phreaker websites are www.phrack.org and www.2600.org, and www.securityfocus.com provides useful information from a security perspective. In addition, most PABX manufacturers provide security information for their products online.

The impact of PABX fraud

Incidents of PABX fraud currently under investigation involve millions of euro, with one injured party incurring in excess of €700 000 in a single loss. Nearly every medium to large institution possesses a PABX, and while these systems offer their users efficiency and flexibility they may also render them vulnerable to attack, and a successful hacker may gain access to the entire network of a company. PABX or telephone fraud frequently involves high cost international and premium rate services, and companies may receive unexpectedly high phone bills within a short period of time.

The two-pronged sting to this type of attack is that the injured party is left with a substantial bill with no redress; details of the culprits are not available from the telecommunications provider. Ordinary businesses operating high tech equipment do not necessarily possess the required expertise in the technology to take advantage of known security or preventive measures, and studies show that companies are frequently reluctant to report the attacks.

At present the legislation to outlaw this type of crime is limited, and the consensus is that most hackers perpetuating PABX fraud are operating from abroad. Therefore it is likely that PABX frauds will continue to flourish and that convictions will remain extremely difficult to obtain. Investigators require specific legislation and better evidence; company records for telecommunications are often insufficient from an investigator's perspective.

8.2.2 Fraud issues in emerging technology

Emerging technologies have facilitated the development of smart end points devices such as smart mobile phones, smart consumer and business landlines, PDAs and miniature PCs with cellular interfaces, etc. Owing to rapid change within the telecommunications industry and continual commercial pressure, there has been a parallel rapid introduction of intelligence on the edges of the networks through corporate voice networks, cellular networks, the PSTN, etc. These changes present law enforcement and regulatory agencies with new challenges. Firstly, the newly deployed technologies have led to the development of end point devices that are effectively PCs, for example:

- Cisco VoIP phones run a normal operating system, and can run third party Java applications;

- the current generation of Nokia phones are capable of running a variety of third party applications and code;

- Compaq IPAQ GPRS;

- the O_2 XDA mobile phone/PDA, which is internet enabled;

- DECT cordless phones, which can send SMS messages over the PSTN.

Therefore an Apache web server could be run on an XDA or a GPRS IPAQ, raising the possibility that these new devices and their descendants will experience the same types of network attack on their applications and code as current PC systems, e.g. buffer overflow exploits. The CSI/FBI Computer Crime and Security survey found that the second most expensive computer crime in 2003 was Denial of Service attacks costing in excess of $65 million (Computer Security Institute, 2003, 2004). Of 445 respondents from 251 organisations, 78 per cent also reported that internet connections are an increasingly frequent point of attack.

If a telecom terminal (rather than a normal PC) is compromised, all the data on the phone – phonebook, call registers, SMS messages, etc. becomes available to the hacker. A compromised Blackberry PDA and mobile (a combined device) could be used to initiate calls, send harassing emails or SMS messages or download illegal data from websites. Denial of service attacks could be the norm, as well as toll fraud attacks.

VoIP technology

VoIP systems are increasingly likely to attract network attacks as fraudsters come to recognise the potential for PSTN toll fraud. At present VoIP infrastructure is eminently attackable as a normal network application, partly because the software implementing VoIP services is often not well written and runs over an unhardened IP infrastructure that is far from perfect (subject to spoofing and sniffing). In addition VoIP is usually operated as part of a normal network by IT staff who are unlikely to possess the expertise required to protect such systems.

Unified messaging systems

Unified messaging systems are systems that deliver voice mail, faxes, emails, etc. to a single integrated system, usually accessible by several channels, e.g. the PSTN and web. There is obvious scope for toll fraud in the way the messages are forwarded, for example emails and faxes can be forwarded to a particular fax number, and voicemails can be sent to a PSTN number etc. The system is only as strong as the user authentication, which can be poor, and may not be adequately understood and implemented by users.

Future developments in telecommunications fraud

These emerging intelligent devices make use of commodity operating systems, applications and code. Therefore, if an exploit for a common handset was developed, attackers could build a sizeable network of zombie phones in the same way that attackers can create a zombie network in order to carry out a network distributed denial of service attack. Once in control of this network of zombie phones, the attackers could, for instance, manipulate telephone votes on TV shows. Zombie phones could be instructed to dial (or SMS) the voting number in order to increase the number of votes cast. Alternatively, a large number of calls could simply overload a particular voting system number, effectively resulting in a denial of service attack; the normal votes received on the other number would guarantee victory.

This type of attack sounds relatively harmless but could become a serious concern if the zombie phones were used for extortion or directed towards important numbers such as the emergency services numbers.

Based on the foregoing, the following trends and developments are foreseeable:

- further legislative changes;
- more proactive policing;
- establishment of specialised investigation teams;
- targeted training of law enforcement officers;
- increased communication between law enforcement agencies.

8.3 The Convention on Cybercrime

The European Commission directives require all member states to enact provisions encouraging legislative harmony and improving cooperation within the European Union, though this presents certain challenges given the different legal systems that exist across the European Union (common law in the UK and Ireland; civil law in all other EU member states).

The harmonising provisions facilitate the operation of extradition treaties within the EU; historically, most treaties required that in order for a person to be extradited (from one jurisdiction to another) a similar offence carrying a minimum punitive provision had to exist in the country from which the person was being extradited. Given the proliferation of the internet and telecommunications systems, the breaching of national borders by criminals using new technology has become widespread, and subsequent investigations have been hampered by law enforcement that only had jurisdiction within the borders of a single nation. It was clear that in order to facilitate investigations, further improvements were required concerning legislative provisions and cooperation, particularly for aspects such as the transfer of evidence and its admissibility across different jurisdictions.

As a number of authors in this book have noted, as a result of the need for greater cooperation, the Council of Europe formulated an international agreement, the Convention on Cybercrime, (Council of Europe, 2001a, 2001b). This provided the basis for countries to harmonise legislation, and more importantly to cooperate in law enforcement. The countries who ratify the Convention agree to implement it in their own domestic legislation and to support the mechanisms for international cooperation which it sets out. The Convention is discussed more fully in Chapter 2.

8.3.1 The Convention and telecommunications crime

For offences relating to telecommunications, the most important section in the Convention is 'Offences against the confidentiality, integrity and availability of computer data and systems', which contains several separate Articles relevant to telecommunications fraud:

- *Article 2* refers to 'illegal access to a computer system' (covered by the Criminal Damage Act 1991 in Ireland).

- *Article 3* refers to 'illegal interception of transmission of computer data'.

- *Article 4* refers to 'data interference' i.e. damage, deletion, alteration etc.

- *Article 5* refers to 'system interference [. . .] the serious hindering [. . .] of the functioning of a computer system'.

- *Article 6* refers to 'misuse of devices', including programs, passwords and similar access controls. Misuse would include committing any of the above offences. Possession or 'making available' these devices is an offence, but only if undertaken 'for the purpose of committing an offence'. This exemption exists to provide for legitimate tools such as vulnerability scanners.

The framework for investigations

Investigations and investigative procedures are addressed in Chapter 2, Section 2 of the Convention. The framework is termed 'procedural law'. The articles that are of significance are Articles 16 to 21, which refer to particular issues as follows:

- Articles 16 and 17 provide for the expedited preservation of computer data (including telecommunications traffic data, i.e. information about the communication and not its content) so that it may be used as evidence in criminal investigations.

- Article 18 requires countries to allow for production orders. These are legal orders (issued to individuals or companies like telecommunications services providers) to disclose data stored on computers, if such data is required as evidence in the investigation of a criminal offence under the Convention.

- Article 19 refers to search and seizure of computer data, providing powers for investigators to search computer systems and to preserve any relevant data found. The article also provides investigators with the powers to compel a person (with knowledge of the system) to provide information to facilitate a search by investigators.

- Articles 20 and 21 refer to the real-time collection of data (such as traffic data), to requests to service providers to collect data, and for the interception of content data.

International cooperation

Chapter 3 of the Convention refers to the framework for international cooperation for cybercrime investigation, and includes:

- Article 24 which addresses extradition.

- Articles 25 to 28 which are concerned with mutual legal assistance in investigations, such as requests by countries to preserve stored data, capture of traffic data or intercept content data, and the seizure of data held on a computer in another country.

- Article 35 requiring the establishment of a 24/7 international central points of contact network, similar to the G8 24/7 contact points (American Bar Association, 2002). This network would be particularly important in relation to arranging mutual legal assistance.

The Convention and telecommunication systems planning

The Convention has recognised the necessity for a unified approach to the investigation of high tech and telecommunications crime in terms of legislative provisions, procedural law and international cooperation.

A key issue arising from the Convention is that it indirectly places obligations on service providers and equipment manufacturers as they will be required to assist investigators. In order to tackle high-tech and telecommunications crime, systems will not only be required to prevent such activity by implementing improved computer security; systems will need to be designed so that investigators are able to collect useful evidence after such crimes have occurred.

This equipment will not only have to collect the evidence – it will also have to comply with forensic computing standards ensuring that any evidence collected will have its integrity maintained, permitting its admissibility in future proceedings. Current log files (while useful) are often designed for system administration and not for intrusion detection or the investigation of crime. Systems operators should be in a position to assist investigations without compromising evidential material. In order to achieve the above objectives it is important to ensure that investigators have the necessary:

1. Awareness of the issues.

2. Training in investigative techniques.

3. Tools to support the investigation in the gathering of admissible evidence.

8.4 Telecommunications investigations

In Europe there are fundamentally two different types of judicial system employed by the member states. The system employed by the Irish and UK justice systems is an 'adversarial' justice system (Doolan, 1999), but an 'inquisitorial' justice system is used by most of the remaining member states of the EU. These differences have implications for the way evidence is collected and presented in courts. In this section we will look at the rules of evidence, its admissibility, explain the concepts of real evidence and hearsay evidence, and discuss digital evidence and digital forensics. The final section explores some of the difficulties encountered in a recent investigation in Ireland.

8.4.1 Evidence

The crux of any criminal proceedings centres round issues of evidence:

- The admissibility of any evidence gathered.
- The interpretation of the evidence presented.

We have used the term evidence on several occasions but the rules of evidence vary from jurisdiction to jurisdiction. Therefore what is admissible as evidence in one jurisdiction may not be admissible in another. Kelleher and Murray (1997) differentiate between the two different types of evidence generated by computers. First, calculations or analyses which are generated by the computer itself are regarded as 'real evidence'. Second, there are documents and records that are held on computer and these are treated as 'hearsay'.

Examples of real evidence are murder weapons, clothes of a victim or items like drugs or firearms found in the possession of an accused. Computers can generate real evidence as suggested above. Kelleher and Murray (1997) discuss the English case R. v. Spiby (91 Cr. App. Rep. 186) in the Court of Criminal Appeal during which it was stated that 'when the information is recorded by mechanical means without the intervention of a human mind, the record made by the machine is admissible in evidence, provided of course, it is accepted that the machine is reliable'. The appellant had been convicted of the unlawful importation of cannabis. The prosecution had used the telephone call logs from the hotel computer to show that a particular guest at that hotel had called the appellant at his home and club. The evidence was deemed to be real evidence and therefore admissible. In this case the computer automatically recorded telephone calls made through the PABX belonging to the hotel. In order for the evidence to be admissible there was an onus on the prosecution to prove that the computer was working properly; the hotel manager gave direct evidence that the machine was working properly and that no one had complained about the bills.

The precise meaning of hearsay evidence is harder to pin down. Consider the following definitions of hearsay evidence as:

- 'An assertion other than one made by a person while giving oral evidence in the proceedings is inadmissible as evidence of any fact or opinion asserted' (Cross, 1990).

- 'Former statements of any person, whether or not he is a witness in the proceedings, may not be given in evidence if the purpose is to tender them as evidence of the truth of the matters asserted in them' (Phipson, 1990).

In layman's terms, a witness may only assert a fact of which he or she is aware or has experienced and second-hand information is inadmissible. For example, Kelleher and Murray (1997) argue that, in the case R. v. Spiby cited above, if the telephone operator had gathered the information that was admitted as evidence and typed it into the computer before it was printed, this would have made it hearsay and therefore inadmissible. There are exceptions to the rule against hearsay which include:

- admissions and confessions of parties;

- dying declarations;

- public documents (e.g. certificates from the register of births, deaths and marriages);

- statements made contemporaneously with an event.

'Digital evidence' is the preferred term for referring to evidence where the characteristic feature of the evidence is that it is digital data. Other terms such as 'computer evidence' and 'electronic evidence' do not accurately describe the full range of digital data that can be adduced as evidence in court proceedings, as they are limited in scope. Some digital evidence may not come from general-purpose computers or from magneto-optical media, e.g. mobile phones have proved to be a valuable source (Willassen, 2003). Digital evidence is now a well established type of evidence and a recent report from an EU project lists around 50 police units dealing with, for example, cybercrime at a national level in 15 EU member states which each have a digital forensics capability (Ó Ciardhuáin and Gillen, 2002).

The Digital Forensics Workshop (Palmer, 2001) gave the following definition for digital forensics:

> The use of scientifically derived and proven methods toward the preservation, collection, validation, identification, analysis, interpretation, documentation and presentation of digital evidence derived from digital sources for the purpose of facilitating or furthering the reconstruction of events found to be criminal, or helping to anticipate unauthorized actions shown to be disruptive to planned operations.

As the definition states, digital forensics refers to the totality of the methods employed in the preservation, analysis and presentation of evidence found on computer media. In the event of proceedings, details concerning the preservation, analysis and presentation of evidence can be given orally to a court by the forensic analyst who performed the examination of the media in question. The forensics analyst appears as a witness and will be subject to cross examination by the defence and may even be required prior to the trial to disclose all evidence found by him or her during the examination. The digital forensic analyst may also be required to have his or her work analysed by an independent or defence analyst to ensure that the process was carried out correctly and that the results are accurate.

8.4.2 Investigation in practice

Probably the most ingenious case of hacking that was recorded in Ireland was perpetrated against the national carrier at the time, Telecom Éireann (now Eircom). In May 1998 the head of Telecom Éireann's card and payphone services section made a complaint to the Gardaí alleging that Telecom Éireann had been defrauded of IR£117 000 by a person or persons unknown who had made calls to a premium rate service (PRS) number 1580 145632, subscribed to Netstar Communications using 'cloned' or simulated call cards.

The services compromised in this attack were premium rate services and the call card public telephone service. The case came to light at the end of April 1998, after a periodic analysis of a database of information on public payphones revealed irregularities; the payphone located at the Howth Road/Dublin Road junction was one of the highest earning payphones in Ireland for the period April 1997 to April 1998, and the bulk of usage on this phone was to premium rate service lines rather than local usage (on average, 60 per cent of usage on a pay phone is local).

The PRS line dialled belonged to the company Netstar Limited and a more detailed analysis of the traffic on this line for March 1998 showed that:

- More than 2500 calls had been made.

- All the calls to the line were from Dublin-based public card phones.

- All calls lasted between 6 and 7 minutes, equivalent to a person using a 100 unit call card.

- The 'on-hook' time between calls was approximately 20 seconds.

- Simultaneous calls were made from different locations.

The Garda investigation also revealed that the suspect company was operating a computer shareware service on the PRS line. This in itself was suspicious as it is extremely unlikely that individuals would look for computer technical support or shareware using a card phone. A search of local advertising media found no advertisements by Netstar promoting their service and when Gardaí called the

PRS from a card phone they found that the telephone was answered automatically and there was a request for a PIN.

In relation to payment flows, the cost of a call to the Netstar Communications PRS line was IR£1.50 per minute. Of this, 96p went to Netstar and the remainder was for VAT payments, Telecom Éireann's share, and a contribution to the funding of the office of Regtel (the Regulator of Premium Rate Services). Each month Telecom Éireann would provide Netstar with a statistics sheet identifying the number and duration of calls in the previous calendar month, and the revenue owed to Netstar by Telecom Éireann. Upon receipt of an invoice from Nestar, Telecom Éireann would forward a cheque to Netstar in full settlement. Due to the sums involved, it was suspected that some illegal activity was occurring, but at this stage it was not clear precisely what it was.

The evidential burden of proof is the 'criminal burden of proof'; the prosecution must prove their case 'beyond a reasonable doubt'. This particular case demonstrates the disproportionate lengths that the investigation team must go to in order to prove their case. A substantial amount of resources in the form of staff time and equipment went in to investigating what ultimately turned out to be a simple case of obtaining money by false pretences (this offence has now been repealed).

Questions

Robin Bryant & Sarah Bryant

1. How is VoIP telecommunication likely to impact upon criminal behaviour?

2. For premium rate calls, which three parties receive a share of the charge paid by the calling customer?

3. How might the internet be involved when a customer is billed for telephone calls they have not intentionally made?

4. What are two motives for PABX fraud, other than to gain access to free calls?

5. What two features render a typical PABX particularly vulnerable to fraud?

6. Why is the Convention on Cybercrime of relevance to the investigation of PABX fraud?

References

American Bar Association (2002) Cyber crime: An International Problem For Every Lawyer, Business & Country. Report published for annual meeting of the American Bar Association in Washington, DC.

Computer Security Institute (2003) 2003 CSI/FBI Computer Crime and Security Survey. CSI 2007 [Online]. Available at: http://www.gocsi.com (Accessed: Oct 12 2007).

Computer Security Institute (2004) 2004 CSI/FBI Computer Crime and Security Survey. CSI 2007 [Online]. Available at: http://www.gocsi.com (Accessed: Oct 12 2007).

Comptroller and Auditor General (2003) Annual Report of the Comptroller and Auditor General, 2002. 1(12): Dublin: The Stationery Office. pp. 155–157.

Council of Europe (2001a) *Convention on Cyber-Crime*. European Treaty Series No. 185. Budapest, Hungary, Nov 23 2001. [Online]. Available at: http://conventions.coe.int/ (Accessed: Oct 12 2007)

Council of Europe (2001b) Explanatory Report on Convention on Cyber-Crime. Strasbourg, France, Nov 8 2001. [Online]. Available at: http://conventions.coe.int/ (Accessed: Oct 12 2007).

Cross, Sir R. (1990) *Cross on Evidence*, 7th edition. London: Butterworths.

Doolan, B. (1999) *Principles of Irish Law*, 5th edition. Dublin: Gill & Macmillan.

Kelleher, D. and Murray, K. (1997) *Information Technology Law in Ireland.* Dublin: Butterworths.

NIST (1999) Common Criteria for Information Technology Security Evaluation, Version 2.1, CCIMB-99-031. 3 parts. US National Institute of Standards and Technology, United States Department of Commerce. August 1999. [Online]. Available at: http://www.cesg.gov.uk/site/ast/biometrics/media/BEM_10.pdf (Accessed: Oct 12 2007).

NIST (2000) PBX vulnerability analysis. Special Publication 800-24. National Institute of Standards and Technology, United States Department of Commerce. August 2000. ISBN 0–7567–2720–0. [Online]. Available at: http://csrc.nist.gov/publications/nistpubs/800–24/sp800–24pbx.pdf (Accessed: Oct 12 2007).

Ó Ciardhuáin, S. and Gillen, P. (2002) Guide to Best Practice in the area of Internet Crime Investigation. Report from EU Falcone Project No. JA1/2001/Falcone/127 *Training: Cyber Crime Investigation – Building a Platform for the Future*. Dublin: An Garda Síochána.

Palmer, G. (2001) A road map for digital forensic research. DFRWS Technical Report DTR-T0001-01 Final, First Digital Forensic Research Workshop, US Air Force Research Laboratory, 6 November 2001. [Online]. Available at: https://www.dfrws.org/2001/dfrws-rm-final.pdf (Accessed: Oct 11 2007).

Phipson, S.L. (1990) *Phipson on Evidence*, 14th edition. London: Sweet & Maxwell.

Telecommunications UK Fraud Forum Training CD Version 1 (2001) [CD ROM]. London, UK: Telecommunications UK Fraud Forum (TUFF).

US Department of Defense (1985) DoD 5200.28-STD, Department of Defense Trusted Computer System Evaluation Criteria. Fort Meade, Maryland, USA: National Computer Security Center.

Willassen, S.Y. (2003) Forensics and the GSM mobile telephone system. *International Journal of Digital Evidence* **2**(1): [Online]. Available at: http://www.utica.edu/ academic/institutes/ecii/publications/articles/A0658858-BFF6-C537– 7CF86A78D6DE746D.pdf (Accessed: Oct 12 2007).

9
Identity and Identity Theft

Angus Marshall and Paul Stephens

At the time of writing, crimes involving identity theft (or, more accurately, identity fraud) have been identified as a major source of loss to the economy, accounting for losses of between £1.3 billion and £1.7 billion in the UK alone (Home Office, 2007).

In order to understand how identity crimes can be committed, particularly through digital means, we need to examine the concept of identity. Although there is a fairly strict mathematical definition of identity as a degree of 'sameness' or 'similarity' between two objects, the use of the word identity to express concepts related to the identification or the recognition of a person can cause some confusion. For the purposes of this discussion therefore, it may be preferable to introduce some other terms to help expand and analyse the concepts; we will consider *identity*, *recognition* and *recognisability*, and *authority* and *authorisation*, and the way these relate to each other.

Note that there are a number of other complementary ways of approaching the definition of identity. For example, Finch suggests that identity is best understood in terms of three facets: personal, social and legal (Finch, 2007). Of the three forms, Finch argues that legal identity (manifested in birth certificates, national insurance numbers and so on) has the greatest primacy and tenacity (Finch, 2007).

Investigating Digital Crime   Edited by Robin Bryant and Sarah Bryant
© 2008 John Wiley & Sons, Ltd

9.1 Concepts of identity

Perhaps the simplest way to start is to consider the everyday concepts of identity and examine how they map into the digital world. A person may meet and recognise dozens of people every day; that person has a mental image of how each other person looks and behaves, and in turn, the majority of these other people each know who he or she is, as separate and distinct individuals. In one of the strict senses of the word, from a philosophical or psychological perspective, the identity of an individual can be considered to be a composite self-perception i.e. it is a mental model which someone has built up of him or herself.

This concept is related to one of the classical tests for intelligence in animals – that of self awareness. If an animal sees itself in a mirror, it can react in one of two ways – either seeing the mirror image as another animal, and reacting appropriately to the threat or chance to mate, or it can exhibit curiosity and show a behavioural pattern which suggests that it is trying to confirm that the reflection is of itself. This behavioural pattern involves the animal moving from side to side, waving its limbs or making other movements as if to check whether the mirror creature will follow. Such an attempt to fool the mirror twin, strongly suggests that the animal is self-aware and has some notion of its own existence in the world. In effect, it has a conception of its own identity.

From the point of view of an individual, identity is thus an awareness of one's own existence in the world, and involves a wide range of factors ranging from being a member of a family, having friends, having a particular job, through to perception of one's own physical traits, behavioural characteristics and likes or dislikes. In this sense, the only person who can really confirm an identity is the actual 'owner' of that identity him or herself. To an external observer, however, a person's 'identity' seems to be a little simpler and the key concept is that of recognition; can we recognise a person?

9.2 Recognition and recognisability

When a person talks about identifying someone or something, he or she is usually referring to a recognition process. Recognition is an inherent task (performed largely automatically by the brain), which helps humans and other animals to interact in communities, and to carry out tasks effectively. Properties of objects (e.g. colour, shape, texture, sound and smell) are associated with each other, forming a collection of attributes, which taken together, enable the viewer to recognise the object as being the same as, or similar to, objects encountered previously. As an example of how this works, consider trying to describe an apple using just one word. Not so easy, but if two, three, four or more words are used the task becomes more straightforward, and as the number of words increases, the accuracy of the description probably increases. As more and more attributes are included, the 'appleness' of the object increases. This is because the internal recognition model for an apple is very complex, containing many attributes, all of which are required to establish that the object in question is really an apple.

So, there are two related, but different concepts; identity, which is a property of an individual and depends on the internal conception held by that individual, and recognition, which is a collection of externally perceivable attributes used collectively to measure degrees of similarity between objects. It is almost impossible to prove someone's identity using the definition of identity described here. Because of the internal nature of this concept of identity, external tests are not sufficient; indeed they may not even be relevant. However, recognition is an easier process to carry out; attributes may be measured until enough have been checked to allow similarity to a known object to be confirmed, and this is the principle upon which biometric passports and ID cards are founded. Thus, the recognition of an object relies on a collection of attributes, or tokens, which allow us (in common parlance) to 'identify' it.

9.2.1 Third party recognition

Consider the situation where recognition needs to be performed, but the person (or object) in question has not been previously encountered. There are really only two options here; either compare its features (or tokens) with those of known persons (or familiar objects) until a close enough match is found, or use a trusted source of information which can provide additional tokens, to enhance the pool of recognition data. The critical factor in the second process is the reliance on a trusted third party to provide the missing data. If the third party cannot be trusted, or is later shown to have been untrustworthy, then the recognition which depends on that third party becomes unreliable.

Where a third party cannot be directly consulted for confirmation of recognition, it becomes necessary to introduce a new mechanism – a trusted token. This can be a password, an action (e.g. a special handshake) or an object which is difficult to obtain and replicate, e.g. a passport. Possession of the trusted token by both parties demonstrates to each party that the other has been in contact with the trusted third party at some time in the past, and that they can, to some extent, trust each other. In addition, they can trust (to some extent) any data associated with the token. For example, a passport showing the name 'George W. Bush' is more inherently believable or trustworthy than a cheap business card with the same name, because of the effort required to obtain an official passport.

This use of a trusted token reflects the way in which the digital world carries out recognition; the process is usually referred to as authorisation or authentication. Digital systems are really not designed to 'mind' about who is using them. Of far more importance is that any person using a system is authorised to use it, and is using it in an approved manner.

9.3 Authority and authorisation

In many everyday situations there is no real need for computer systems (or indeed people) to be able to recognise a person attempting to carry out a task. The real challenge lies in demonstrating that the person has the authority (permission) to perform the actions required.

This authority can be granted in many ways, ranging from possession of a trusted token, through to personal recognition of the individual in question by a guardian, a person charged with protecting a critical resource. Historically, for example, it has been reported that the easiest way to steal a billiards table from a pub is arrive in a suitable lorry wearing a high visibility jacket and carrying a clipboard. By dressing in an appropriate manner and acting confidently, the criminal can assume an air of authority which is difficult to challenge. The guardian believes that they recognise the category of person who has come to collect the billiards table as appropriate, and allows it to be taken away.

People are, in effect, conditioned to expect that people dressed in a particular way (and who behave in a congruent manner) have the authority to carry out certain actions, without needing any further proof of their authority. Effectively then, in certain circumstances, for police officers, soldiers, sailors, doctors and nurses, the clothes really do 'maketh the man' (or woman) and are often the only trusted token required to allow certain activities.

9.4 Recognition and authority in the digital world

Digital devices generally have extremely limited recognition ability and tend to depend wholly on the presence of trusted tokens. These tokens, provided initially by system administrators, take many forms, but the most common tend to use a two-factor authentication approach.

9.4.1 *n*-factor authentication

In mathematics, the letter n is used to denote any number. Therefore n-factor authentication refers to the number of components required to show that the trusted token being presented is valid.

A one factor authentication scheme employs a single token. A single factor (such as a uniform) is required to establish authority, with no further confirmation or challenge. It is inherently a weak system because the authority lies wholly with possession of just one token; there is no requirement to attempt to establish that the person presenting the token has obtained it legitimately and truly has the right to use that token. Consider the situation where a computer terminal is asking for a user to log on to the system. Simply accepting that any person who types in the log-in name 'Gordon Brown' is an authorised person, without further challenge, is probably not the best way to control access to the launch codes for the UK's nuclear missiles. One factor authentication is, therefore, not generally considered adequate as a measure for establishing authority, because of the scope for easy forgery and lying.

The most commonly deployed system is a two-factor authentication scheme. These usually operate on a present-challenge-response system; the user presents an initial component and is then challenged to respond with a second confirmatory component. In computer systems, this usually takes the form of a username and password procedure. For banking, a plastic card bearing a unique number is used (the initial component), coupled with either a PIN (personal identification number) or signature, or a CVV (cardholder verification value) for transactions where the cardholder is not present (see Chapter 7 for further details). The underlying principle is that while it is relatively easy to acquire a single component, it is harder to obtain two tokens, particularly as the two tokens need to be compatible.

Beyond two-factor authentication, more complex authentication systems require more components in order to carry out the recognition process, making it increasingly difficult for unauthorised users to acquire sufficient trusted tokens to be recognised by the system. Some of these tokens may be abstract such as a username and password, while others may be physical objects or images such as fingerprints or a retinal scan. A variation on n-factor authentication requires that a user has access to a pool of trusted tokens, and the authentication system requests a random subset of these, limiting the number of tokens disclosed at any one time. The advantage of this method is that it reduces the possibility that an eavesdropper will be able to gain access to a valid pool of tokens; even if an eavesdropper manages to copy all of the tokens used to gain access for one particular session, the subsequent session is likely to require production of a different subset, so the impersonation will fail.

9.5 Obtaining information through social engineering

Social engineering is a relatively new term, encompassing a number of related ideas, all emphasising the importance of the human element in the transfer of trusted tokens from one person to another, particularly in relation to identity theft and fraud. If a victim is tricked or persuaded into divulging personal information, this is a clear-cut case of social engineering. However, the term is also used to describe a wider range of scenarios, including any circumstances that exploit the lack of awareness or naivety of a victim, such as dustbin sifting; some householders are unaware that certain items of paperwork in domestic rubbish is of potential criminal use. Inevitably, some activities may include only a small element of social engineering, and for these reasons it is not possible to formulate a clear-cut definition of social engineering. It is clear that the term is used in a variety of ways, and refers to a range of practices.

Techniques for obtaining personal information from a 'mark' (victim) range from the low-tech, such as sifting through rubbish (or dumpster diving as it is known in the US), to methods that have traditionally been associated with crackers, such as Trojan horses. This section outlines some of the main ways of obtaining information through exploiting the human element of a system.

The reformed hacker Kevin Mitnick stresses the importance of the human element in security and is largely responsible for popularising the term social engineering. In his first book *The Art of Deception: Controlling the Human Element of Security*, he claims that '[...] I could often get passwords and other pieces of sensitive information from companies by pretending to be someone else and just asking for it [...] the human factor is truly security's weakest link.' (Mitnick and Simon, 2002, p. 3).

9.5.1 Persuasion, manipulation and bribery

Persuasion is a broad term encompassing a wide range of social interactions, from pleasurable and witty flirtatiousness to bribery, violence and blackmail. Many types of persuasion involve some level of deceit, and the victim may concur with the deceit if they find the interaction gratifying in some way. Persuasion can be especially effective if the attacker helps the victim to develop a sense of empathy. The victim gains a sense of well-being from the exchange and is likely to become more trusting and less cautious. In this state of mind, a victim is more likely to reveal personal information on request.

Many social engineering attacks rely on the attacker deceiving the victim as to the attacker's true identity; for example, the social engineer could pose as an authority figure. There is often a hint of implied threat concerning the repercussions of such an exchange, particularly if the authority figure appears dissatisfied. In this case, fear rather than pleasure is used to persuade a victim to divulge information.

Lastly, bribery can be employed as a means of persuasion. This does not necessarily mean meeting in multi-storey car parks in raincoats and dark glasses, handing over brown envelopes stuffed with £50 notes. Organisers of Infosecurity Europe 2003 found that many office workers were willing to give away their computer passwords for a cheap pen (Leyden, 2003). The same group in 2004 found that over 70 per cent of people revealed their password for a chocolate bar (BBC, 2004). The same survey found that 79 per cent of people interviewed gave details that could be used to commit identity theft. The 2007 survey found that 64 per cent of people were willing to give their password (Skinner, 2007). Whilst some of the respondents were almost certainly lying in exchange for a small gift, many people do regularly give away personal details to surveys and salespeople, both in the street and over the telephone.

9.5.2 Help desk attacks

Help desk attacks tend to take one of two forms. The first is that of phoning a help desk and requesting information, hoping to persuade the call handler to reveal information. Although directly requesting information may work, quite often the attacker may use a more sophisticated approach. For example, if a fictional social engineer, Dave, wanted to find out about a company's network, he could try the following:

Dave: *Hi, my name's Dave Lightman. I'm a salesman for Matrix Computer Solutions. I got a call from Bob Cratchit* [name of someone in the computer department perhaps gleaned from the company website, unlikely to be available as it is lunchtime] *and he was interested in some of our firewall solutions.*

Call-handler:	Hi, you've actually come through to the help desk and he's probably at lunch at the moment.
Dave:	*Oh, right . . . this is the number he left . . . I wonder if you could give me his number?*
Call-handler:	Sure, his number is 123456
Dave:	*Excellent! Thanks ever so much. I don't suppose you could give me some information before I speak to him . . . it was quite a garbled message I got and I don't want to look like an idiot?*
Call-handler:	Um, OK.

At this stage Dave could ask some further more probing questions, such as what exactly Bob Cratchit's role at the company is and whether he controls the budget. He could then move on to ask about the number of PCs on the network, the type of network, and the operating systems used by the web server. Social engineers tend to be skilled at building up a sense of camaraderie with a mark. They may make themselves seem naive so that they seem innocuous, and some questions they ask may be used to build up a false sense of security in the victim.

The second form of help desk attack relies on the customer's lack of awareness, combined with their likely respect for authority. The attacker simply eavesdrops on the victim's interaction, for example at a bank help desk; the bank clerk will often ask personal questions such as date of birth and mother's maiden name to ascertain customer identity. Many customers may feel uneasy, but at the same time do not wish to appear rude or 'difficult', so provide the information in a rather too public setting.

To help companies to avoid the first kind of attack, a programme of training concerning the risks of social engineering could be introduced, as well as some well-defined policies regarding the dissemination of potentially sensitive information. Individuals wanting to avoid the second attack would be well advised to stand their ground, (or not to shout too loudly, no matter how big a mistake the bank has made). Discretion is definitely the better part of valour when giving out personal information.

9.5.3 Phishing

Phishing is a technique used to obtain trusted tokens such as usernames, passwords, and other sensitive personal data, such as credit card details and PIN numbers. The attacker usually sends a large number of emails claiming to be

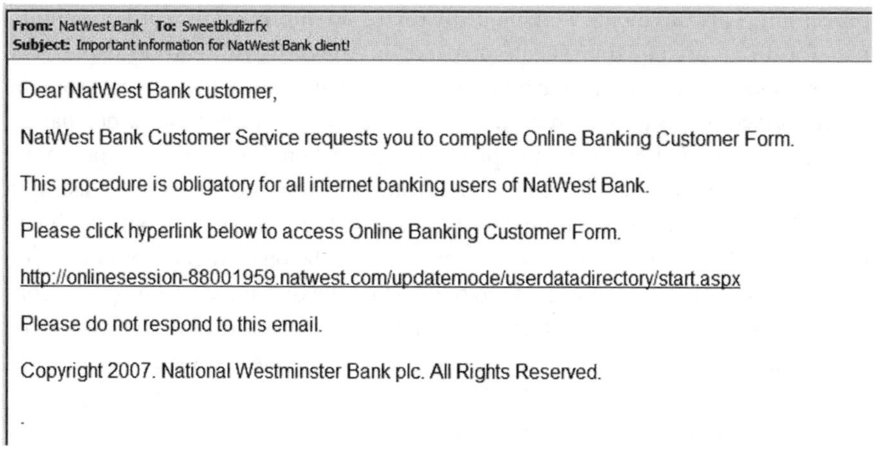

From: NatWest Bank   **To:** Sweetbkdlizrfx
Subject: Important information for NatWest Bank client!

Dear NatWest Bank customer,

NatWest Bank Customer Service requests you to complete Online Banking Customer Form.

This procedure is obligatory for all internet banking users of NatWest Bank.

Please click hyperlink below to access Online Banking Customer Form.

http://onlinesession-88001959.natwest.com/updatemode/userdatadirectory/start.aspx

Please do not respond to this email.

Copyright 2007. National Westminster Bank plc. All Rights Reserved.

Figure 9.1   An unsophisticated attempt at phishing

from any organisation that might have access to, or require a customer's financial details, for example, a customer's bank or ISP. Figure 9.1 shows a typical attempt at phishing. Note the clumsy wording and the unconvincing URL for the hypertext link.

The email will claim that for some reason, such as a 'system up-date', customer information is required and that the victim should follow the link in the email to verify account details. The linked website is another forgery, set up by the attacker, and it stores the details entered by the victim. Both the email received and the linked website can appear to be completely genuine. Customers of popular online banks and users of PayPal and eBay are often the target of this kind of attack.

It may seem difficult to appreciate why many people share personal information in such an unguarded way, however, even in the early days of the development of computer technology one can find examples of intelligent software programs which have been able to elicit very personal private information from individuals (Weizenbaum, 1966). The latest version of Microsoft Internet Explorer, Mozilla Firefox, and Opera contain anti-phishing features. The use of spam filters for email accounts may also reduce the likelihood of receiving phishing messages.

9.5.4 'Dumpster diving'

Historically, some of the earliest effective methods of obtaining financial tokens lie in the early days of credit cards. Prior to the introduction of online payment processing, card payments were made by taking an imprint of the card on a multi-part form comprising four sheets of paper interleaved with carbon paper. The customer kept one copy and the retailer kept the others to obtain payment from the credit card company and as a record of the transaction. However, the carbon papers were not required after the card imprint had been taken. It became common practice for the carbon papers to be removed from the imprinted vouchers and simply discarded. At the end of a trading day, the discarded carbon papers would be tipped into a waste bin, skip or 'dumpster' along with all the other waste from the store.

Inevitably, criminals soon came to realise that the discarded carbon paper contained complete copies of all the information on the card plus a copy of the cardholder's signature. Thus by spending a few minutes or even a few hours dumpster diving a fraudster could obtain copies of all the cards which had passed through the store that day. With a little bit of effort a perfect copy of the embossed plastic card could be produced and, the fraudster could copy and learn to reproduce the cardholder's signature. Thus the possession of two tokens (card and signature) could be used to subsequently gain authority over the cardholder's account. Alternatively, by simply placing a telephone order (relying on just a single token – the card number), further purchases could be made.

This mechanism, of course, exploited a major flaw in the payment handling system – the carbon papers. As soon as online payment authorisation became available, using data held on the magnetic stripe on the back of the card, this option started to disappear and a new challenge was faced. Although dumpster diving no longer really works for credit card fraud, it can still be used effectively for the type of fraud noted above – personal information in the form of bank and credit card statements, bills, personal letters, etc. are regularly discarded with domestic and business waste. A little bit of time spent rooting through rubbish can yield sufficient data to commit fraud. The problem of dustbin sifting has been well publicised in the UK and many high street shops and supermarkets sell shredders making the sifter's task much more difficult.

9.5.5 Web browsing

Social networking sites such as Facebook, Bebo and MySpace have received negative publicity recently (BBC, 2007) as they have been used to collect information which could subsequently provide key trusted token components of a false identity. Social networkers post a variety of personal details on these sites, including the kind of information used by financial institutions to verify a person's identity. Although social networking sites are currently the focus of attention, all websites containing personal information could be subject to the same criticism. This includes company websites that give biographical details and online CVs.

The simple solution to this problem is to exclude any personal information from any website, but this undermines the purpose of many of these sites; most people using social networking sites enjoy sharing information, including personal information. The majority of social networking sites allow users to restrict the availability of information, and to specify who may view it. Some users blatantly lie in answer to some of the questions, to provide some element of protection against unscrupulous use of personal details. For example, when answering questions about how friends first met, decoy answers such as 'Attending drug rehabilitation in 1978' or 'Flying in Tanzania' are likely to reduce the value of other personal information posted on sites, and to confuse an impersonator. Poor information can be just as bad as no information, and indeed the replication of false information in a false identity profile may help an investigator trace the source of the false details. To avoid criminal exploitation, users should certainly not use published personal information as answers to any security or password questions.

9.6 ID Fraud in practice

Accepting the definitions above leads to the conclusion that the activity usually called 'ID Theft' or 'ID Fraud' can be more accurately considered to be 'Authority Fraud'. The criminal seeks to obtain authority to carry out some action (which they are not, in reality, permitted to perform) by acquiring sufficient tokens to convince someone or something that they are a legitimate user of the service and hence authorised to use it.

The criminal's aim is not to break the system and bypass security, nor to force it to accept invalid tokens, but simply to exploit an inherent weakness in the authority-granting mechanism, a mechanism which relies on trust in the user being established through the presence of sufficient tokens. If the number of tokens is small or the security surrounding the tokens is low (e.g. easily guessed passwords, data which can be found from public sources) and the acquired trust level is high, the damage can be great. So, for the criminal, the challenge lies in the acquisition of the tokens themselves.

9.6.1 Jackals and data aggregators

In Frederick Forsyth's novel *The Day of the Jackal* a mechanism is described for obtaining a passport in a false name. The method employed involves establishing the identity of a person who has died and then using public offices to obtain copies of official documents (e.g. birth certificate) which can be used to create sufficient trust to allow official bodies (in the Jackal's case, a passport office) to issue official documents. In this way, the fraudster assumes the identity of the deceased person. Because the Jackal's false passport was issued by an official passport office, it would pass all tests for validity and have a very high trust value.

The Jackal's process was relatively high-risk because it involved personal visits to government offices to obtain the necessary documents. He needed to see records of births and deaths and submit forms in person. In the modern world, much of this data (e.g. electoral registers, telephone directories, property registers) must be made available to the public, and although it can still be viewed at official buildings, it is also available online – convenient for the innocent member of the public and the fraudster alike.

In addition, data from several of these sources are collated by a variety of companies to produce aggregated data sets from which further information can be deduced. For example, some websites allow telephone numbers to be associated with a named individual at a specific address. In a telephone directory, this would usually be limited to the telephone subscriber, but by combining telephone directory data with electoral registers, it is possible for a data aggregator to associate the phone number with any person over the age of 18 at the subscribers address. Furthermore, by storing electoral register details over several years, changes in relationships (e.g. marriage, divorce, death) and ages (e.g. above or below the voting age) can be deduced.

Data aggregation sites such as these have been used in the past by criminals to obtain 'loans', or more accurately, considerable sums of money as they are never repaid. By searching property registers, telephone directories and electoral registers, families are identified who have:

- changed address recently; and

- applied for unsecured loans.

The standard requirement for such an application requires the applicant to have had the same address for at least 2 years, or to have been at their previous address for a similar period of time. The fraudster searches for new entries on a property register, and thereby selects a person who has recently moved house; this person is now the target. The criminal then finds the target's previous address from telephone directories and electoral registers. The criminal then applies for a loan in the target's name, claiming to have recently moved to the criminal's chosen false address (often only used for the duration of the fraud). However, as part of the application for the loan, the criminal gives a false previous address, providing the target's previous address instead.

Because the credit reference files consulted by the financial institutions are based on historical data, the target's name (being used fraudulently by the criminal) is associated with the previous address. The credit records for the target are reasonable, and the company is fooled into believing it has a legitimate application from a low-risk applicant. The loan is granted and the criminal receives the payment at his or her chosen address.

Of course, the criminal has no intention of repaying the loan, and as the lender has no real clue to their identity (and has a false address), the criminal is more than likely to get away with the scam. This type of activity may go undetected for some considerable time as the target whose identity is being used fraudulently is unlikely to be aware of the activity. The target has no way of knowing, because all the documents and communications concerning the loan will be directed to the criminal's chosen address.

The tokens used by the criminal are all a matter of public record. This may (after considering the fraud described above) seem unnecessarily risky, but it can be (and has been) argued that such information must be in the public domain in order to prevent fraud (e.g. in elections and property deals), as well as ensuring that information such as telephone numbers are available for the general convenience of the public. Note that no physical tokens are used, only information.

In all cases, the aim of the ID fraudster is the same – to obtain sufficient tokens, usually in the form of personal data, to enable a fraudster to convince a third party that he or she is a legitimate account holder, loan applicant, member of staff or other authorised person. Exact methods vary, but all tend to rely on an existing trust relationship (customer to waiter/waitress, customer to bank, employee to employer, etc.) in which data are regularly disclosed or inappropriate disposal of sensitive data. The key to identifying the precise point at which the fraud began, is to identify the point at which the data first escaped from the trusted environment and was acquired by the criminal.

9.7 Investigating identity theft

In the UK several strategies have been adopted by the government and its agencies in an attempt to prevent identity theft. There is an increased focus on deterrence through harsher penalties, including:

- defining new criminal offences relating to identity fraud with additional legislation (e.g. The Identity Cards Act 2006 and The Fraud Act 2006);

- increasing penalties associated with fraudulently obtaining certain documents (e.g. The Criminal Justice Act 2003).

The government has also sought to make it more difficult to obtain documents fraudulently by:

- introducing more stringent measures to obtain a passport (e.g. an interview for first-time applicants);

- increasing collaboration and dissemination of information between financial institutions, passport agencies and driving licence issuers; and

- raising public awareness of the problem of identity theft (Home Office, 2007).

The emphasis seems to be on the prevention of the crime; investigation tends to be time consuming and labour intensive. Indeed, the UK's Fraud Prevention Service, Cifas, claims that it 'is estimated that the police investigate less than 1 % of identity fraud cases' (Cifas, 2005) although the evidence to support this is not provided on their website. In October 2007, the House of Commons All Party Parliamentary Group on Identity Fraud recommended that police forces appoint identity fraud officers with a specific remit for investigating identity theft related offences.

There are several ways in which an investigation can proceed. Identity fraud is not an end in itself; the aim of the perpetrator is often financial gain, or obtaining goods or services. The acquisition processes inevitably leave a paper trail which may include forged signatures and photocopies of illegally obtained documents. Other documents, such as those used for mail order goods and document delivery may provide evidence of addresses and mobile phone numbers used by the suspect. If items are bought in person then CCTV footage might provide photographic evidence, such as images of the suspect.

If enough evidence is collected then a search of the suspect's address could be legally justified. This might include some dustbin sifting by the law enforcement officers themselves.

Questions

Robin Bryant & Sarah Bryant

1. In what ways has the internet assisted those who wish to steal others' identity?

2. What technological measures are available to counter identity theft? How effective are they likely to be?

3. How is social engineering facilitated through the use of the internet?

4. Some online banking sites require just three of the six digits from a customer's passnumber to access an account online. How can the use of three digits (rather than six) enhance the security of the customer's online account?

5. You move house, and forget to inform your bank. In what ways might this leave you vulnerable to fraud?

References

BBC (2004) Passwords revealed by sweet deal. BBC News [Online]. Available at: http://news.bbc.co.uk/1/hi/technology/3639679.stm (Accessed: Aug 2 2007).

BBC (2007) Web networkers 'at risk of fraud'. BBC News [Online]. Available at: http://news.bbc.co.uk/1/hi/uk/6910826.stm (Accessed: Aug 1 2007).

Cifas (2007) Is identity theft serious? BBC News [Online]. Available at: http://www.cifas.org.uk/default.asp?edit_id=556–56 (Accessed: Oct 11 2007).

Finch, E. (2007) The problem of stolen identity. (Chapter 3). In: Y. Jewkes (ed.) *Crime Online*. Cullompton: Willan Publishing, pp. 29–43.

Home Office (2007) Home Office Identity Theft Steering Committee. [Online]. Available at: http://www.identity-theft.org.uk/faqs.html (Accessed: Sep 4 2007).

Leyden, J. (2003) Office workers give away passwords for a cheap pen. [Online]. Available at: http://www.theregister.co.uk/2003/04/18/office_workers_give_away_passwords/ (Accessed: Aug 2 2007).

Mitnick, K.D. and Simon, W.L. (2002) *The Art of Deception: Controlling the Human Element of Security*. Indianapolis: Wiley Publishing, Inc.

Skinner, C. (2007) Two-thirds tell you their password for a bar of chocolate. [Online]. Available at: http://www.finextra.com/community/fullblog.aspx?id=176 (Accessed: Aug 2 2007).

Weizenbaum, J. (1966) ELIZA – A computer program for the study of natural language communication between man and machine, *Communications of the ACM* **9**(1):35–36.

10

Internet Grooming and Paedophile Crimes

Denis Edgar-Nevill

It is often difficult to understand many forms of criminal activity, particularly those that involve exploiting and abusing the weak or vulnerable, and crimes against children in particular, especially those which involve sexual acts, evoke very strong emotions in the general population. Crimes against children are not new, but digital technology now provides powerful access mechanisms and new opportunities for such crimes to be committed.

One positive aspect of the modern age is a more open, less stigmatized feeling amongst the victims of paedophiles, resulting in a crop of prosecutions for offences committed in the last half of the twentieth century. Victims now feel more able to divulge what happened, including events which occurred many years previously, and to bring prosecutions. In July 2007 the Roman Catholic Church in Los Angeles settled cases with 508 victims of child abuse by clergy, with a total pay out of $660 million (brought at 15 legal actions). Some of the cases concerned incidents occurring as long ago as the 1940s (BBC, 2007; USA Today, 2007).

Investigating Digital Crime   Edited by Robin Bryant and Sarah Bryant
© 2008 John Wiley & Sons, Ltd

10.1 Pre-digital paedophile crime

Myra Hindley and Ian Brady were convicted in 1966 of the 'Moors Murders'; so named because four of the victims were buried on Saddleworth Moor between Lancashire and West Yorkshire. Brady was convicted of the murder of three children (John Kilbride, Lesley Ann Downey, and Edward Evans) and subsequently confessed to two further murders (Pauline Reade and Keith Bennett) in prison in 1987. Hindley was convicted of the murder of two of the victims (Lesley Ann Downey, and Edward Evans). It is widely believed that there was a sexual motive for these abductions and murders.

The distribution of child pornography also predates modern technology. For example, in 1974 the 'Paedophile Information Exchange' (PIE) was formed in the UK. It initially communicated with members through a newsletter and later with a magazine called 'Understanding Paedophilia', which in part attempted to provide an academic justification of paedophile activity. It was eventually replaced with the magazine 'Magpie', which altered the format to include articles, clothed photographs of children, jokes about paedophilia and letters from the members of PIE. Five PIE members were charged in 1978 with printing contact advertisements calculated to promote indecent acts between adults and children and in 1981 Tom O'Carroll (a former chairman of PIE) was convicted on a conspiracy charge and sentenced to two years in prison. In 1984 there were further successful prosecutions for possession of child pornography involving PIE members; PIE was disbanded in 1984.

10.2 The internet and paedophile crimes

The facilitation of paedophile activity is one of the more negative aspects of the communication revolution brought about by the internet. The origins of the internet can be traced back to the development of ARPANET in the 1960s and 1970s (Hauben, 2007) but it did not become the all-pervasive facility we use today until the development of the World Wide Web (WWW) in 1989 (CERN, 1989). Before the development of the WWW, the internet was mainly used for text communication by email, without an attachment facility; it was technically possible to exchange pictures but this was not without difficulty. The WWW was a veritable revolution, providing a simple and accessible means of displaying pictures and text together, as in a printed book or magazine. With the ability to see pictures came the explosive growth of internet usage around the World. Over the past 15 years or so, the internet has approximately doubled in size every year (Coffman and Odlyzko, 2001) so over 10 years it has increased in size by a factor in excess of 1000; the accessibility of adult pornography in western Europe is regarded as a significant driver in the growth of websites and number of people accessing the WWW.

In the 1990s, adult pornography sites were less sophisticated and less driven by subscription and financial reward than today. It was as if all the top-shelf pornographic publications in newsagents were suddenly put onto the bottom shelf and were being given away free to anyone of any age. In recent years many search engines, including Yahoo, have made considerable efforts to address the problem by restricting access and by filtering search terms, however it is difficult to devise such a procedure that will not inadvertently prevent users accessing informative and harmless sites.

10.3 A brief history

This section provides an overview of the most significant police investigations into child internet pornography.

In 1998 over 100 men were detained in 'Operation Cathedral', involving police raids in the UK, USA, Australia, Belgium, Finland, Austria, Germany, France, Norway, Italy, Portugal and Sweden. In total, 750 000 images and 1800 digital movies were seized. Twelve of the men arrested were from the UK; nine faced charges resulting from their arrests and eight were eventually convicted and received prison sentences ranging from 12 to 30 months.

'Operation Avalanche' took place in Texas in 1999. A member of the public tipped off the Dallas Police about a website advertising child pornography. The website was investigated with the help of Microsoft and traced to an internet gateway and credit clearance company; Landslide Inc. The company's owners, Thomas and Janice Reedy, were arrested, and police seized a database listing over 45 000 subscribers, mainly from the US, UK and Canada. Thomas and Janice Reedy were offered prison terms of 20 years and 5 years respectively if they agreed to cooperate with the investigation; they refused, and Thomas Reedy was sentenced in 2001 to 1335 years in prison (reduced to 180 years on appeal) after being found guilty of 89 charges involving sexual exploitation of minors and distribution of child pornography. The true scale of the operation included more than 250 000 subscribers and provided access to 5700 different websites around the World (BBC, 2001), with a turnover of $1.4m a month. In the US, the credit card records led to 144 searches in 37 US states. The existence of Operation Avalanche was made public in 2001, following the first prosecutions resulting from the Landslide Inc records.

'Operation Ore' began in 1999 as the UK arm of Operation Avalanche. The Landslide Inc. names and credit card details were made available by US authorities, leading to 3744 arrests in the UK. However, many of the people arrested had had no links with child pornography but had instead been victims of credit card fraud and identity theft; the resulting protests and legal actions cast a shadow over the whole investigation (Sheriff, 2007).

Of particular interest to the media in the UK was the case in 1999 involving the pop star Gary Glitter; his computer was found to contain approximately 4000 stored images of child abuse. He pleaded guilty and was convicted in June 2006, and his appeal against a conviction for molesting three young girls at his villa in Vietnam was rejected (Billboard, 2006). While there is no suggestion that internet grooming was involved, clearly the development of computer technology is likely to have facilitated his development as a paedophile; this technology was unavailable even a decade before.

Child Pornography Offenders

Robin Bryant

A key research and practical question is the relationship between the use of child pornography and sexual offending against children by adults. These are difficult and uncomfortable questions but it does not necessarily follow that a person who accesses child pornography for fantasy (usually masturbatory) reasons would, by necessity, be involved in (or become involved in) physical sexual abuse of children. Of course it can be argued that the use of child pornography alone (even so-called computer generated pseudo images) creates a demand for this 'product' which in turn leads to harm against children. Nonetheless it is important, if only in terms of the deployment of limited police resources, that individuals' motives for using child pornography are better understood. Krone (2004) listed nine different types of offender associated with child pornography online. Figure 10.1 below summarises his typology (Krone's categories are shown in bold) and the possible links between types of behaviour and offending. The dotted lines show probable development routes from one category to another.

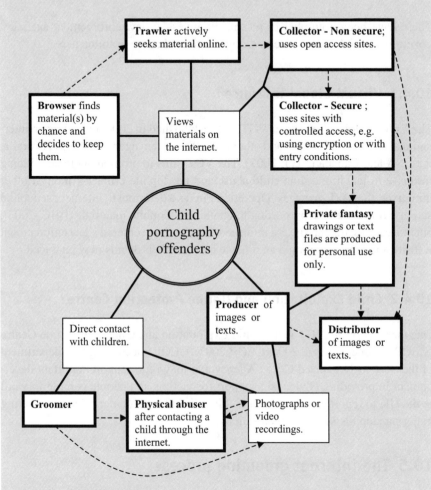

Figure 10.1 A typology of online child pornography offenders

Reference

Krone, T. (2004) *A Typology of Online Child Pornography Offending*. [Online]. Available at: http://www.aic.gov.au/publications/tandi2/tandi279.pdf. (Accessed: Oct 22 2007).

10.4 Recent initiatives to combat internet child pornography

There have been a number of recent initiatives, by law enforcement agencies, governments and other concerned organisations that we examine here.

10.4.1 Virtual Global Taskforce

The Virtual Global Taskforce (VGT) was established in 2004, providing an international alliance of Interpol and other law enforcement agencies across Australia, the USA and Canada (VGT, 2007). The VGT aims to promote a global policing response to tackling online child abuse and paedophile crimes. Amongst other initiatives, the VGT manages 'Operation Pin' as a deterrent to internet paedophile activity. It is a website purporting to contain paedophile materials (BBC, 2003), but those accessing the site are informed that they have entered a law enforcement website and have committed an offence and that their details may be traced.

10.4.2 Child Exploitation and Online Protection Centre

One member of the VGT is the Child Exploitation and Online Protection Centre (CEOP), formed in April 2006 (CEOP, 2007). CEOP is a cross agency department of the Serious Organised Crime Agency and may represent an important development in providing advice and support for victims and people coming forward in the UK to report crimes against children. It has a particular role in combating major paedophile support organisations.

10.5 The internet grooming process

Grooming is the deliberate cultivation of a relationship for an ulterior and undisclosed motive, and usually involves an older person befriending a younger or vulnerable person. If grooming takes place using the internet, it is easy for the groomer to deceive their victim; for instance, many groomers claim to be much younger than they are in reality, and befriend children or adolescents.

The study of a number of criminal cases of internet grooming suggest a common sequence of stages through which this process might pass and will be further discussed in the following sections. A summary of the stages is given in figure 10.2.

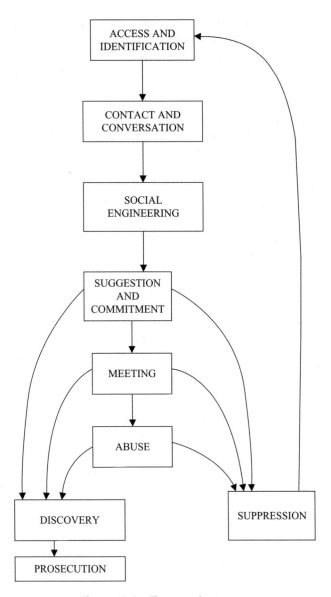

Figure 10.2   The grooming process

10.5.1 Access

Gaining access to someone has never been easier. The internet provides practically unrestricted electronic access to more than 1.1 billion people, including children. Groomers no longer have to physically stalk potential victims; instead from the privacy of their own homes they can use a variety of cheap and accessible internet communications mechanisms to contact potentially millions of children:

- *Email* – freely accessible and comparatively anonymous (Qi and Edgar-Nevill, 2007); the oldest form of communication on the internet;

- *Newsgroups and other forums* – posting and sharing communications on particular subjects with groups of users;

- *Chat rooms* – online discussion forums for meeting and holding a conversation, visible to other users who have joined the chat room. The conversations which take place may be moderated by a person in the room; the moderator can warn and even ban users who communicate inappropriately;

- *Instant messaging services* – one-to-one real-time message exchanges between users. Many sites have instant messaging as a by-product of the purpose of the site. For example, Yahoo Chess includes a chat area for players to communicate (and users are given warning messages about their potential misuse).

In the last few years, Web 2.0 has been associated with a significant increase in the number of social networking websites. Internet users have felt increasingly empowered to use the internet for personal communication, as well as for sourcing information. Web 2.0 is not a new piece of software; the term Web 2.0 (first used in 2003 by O'Reilly Associates (O'Reilly Associates, 2007)) merely indicates a more interactive and user-led style of internet use.

Web 2.0 is associated with developments such as:

- blogs (e.g. Blogger, 2007);

- wikis (e.g. Wiki, 2007);

- profiles (e.g. MySpace, 2007);

- pictures (e.g. Flickr, 2007);

- digital video (e.g. YouTube, 2007);

- preferences (e.g. Del.icio.us, 2007).

At the time of writing it seems likely that Web 2.0 may inadvertently also provide a basis and mechanism for paedophile crime and many other forms of crime (such as identity theft), partly because users of facilities willingly share so much information about themselves.

10.5.2 Identification

A groomer selects or identifies a victim, and there are particular advantages for the groomer if this is carried out over the internet. Because of the private and personal nature of communication with a machine, it is much easier for some people to build friendships and personal relationships online. It is possible that an otherwise isolated person may be more likely to be attracted by online invitations to share relationships.

Any person who is unaware of the possibility of deception is inevitably more vulnerable to deception. New facilities come online practically every day, and many home computer users may be unaware of the novel ways in which they might be deceived. For example, large numbers of home computers are hijacked to act as zombie slaves to rebroadcast spam emails hiding their true source.

Wi-fi access in homes has made it easy to set up computers with internet links in bedrooms and so an increasing number of children now have their own computer in their own room, leading to an inevitable decrease in the level of supervision by parents or other carers. A child with low level of supervision is clearly more vulnerable to grooming.

10.5.3 Contact and conversation

The point at which first contact is made is important for a number of reasons:

1. It may be the start of a trail of evidence that might be important in any future prosecution;

2. The precise number of communications between the groomer and victim may determine if the crime of internet grooming has been committed in law (Sexual Offences Act 2003);

3. The first contact might be consequent to the commission of other offences, such as unauthorised access (Computer Misuse Act 1990) or a previous offender breaking the terms or conditions of their release from custody;

4. Establishing when the first contact occurred may be important in providing evidence for investigations relating to other victims. For example, there is growing evidence that many internet groomers initially contact many potential victims within a short time, but pursue conversations with only the most promising.

For a groomer, the internet has many advantages, including the opportunity to assume a 'cyber-identity', disguising their own age, gender, ethnicity or location. A groomer might pretend to be a child; perhaps the same age as the victim or, more usually, one or two years older. Evidence of an assumed identity can be an important factor in establishing that a series of communications constitutes grooming.

A key part of establishing a dialogue is to persuade the potential victim to reply to a directed message; possibly to a question about something innocuous. At this stage, the conversation is likely to be taking place in the view of other users; in a public chat room or messaging facility. However, the groomer will be aiming to move the conversation to a more private space on a one-to-one basis in a private chat room or instant message facility. The conversation might then be developed to the point where the victim communicates over repeated log-ins, times and days. All of these communications build up a body of evidence that might be used in a prosecution as evidence of intent; a key feature of grooming.

There is some evidence from criminal cases to suggest that groomers try not to prolong communications, possibly as a means of restricting the volume of evidence. If an investigator has access to a whole series of communications containing suggestions made in different ways, the overall tone and direction of the interaction is likely to be clearer. However, it is much more difficult to demonstrate unequivocal intent from one short email; the interpretation might be dependent on the meaning of just a few individual ambiguous words or phrases.

10.5.4 Social engineering and internet grooming

Starting with only a little information, a groomer might access internet sources to begin building a fuller profile of their victim. The victim may subsequently be impressed if the groomer knows even small incidental snippets of information, and consequently be persuaded to disclose more sensitive information. Children can be very trusting, particularly if another person appears to know much about them, their family, or their state of mind.

Communication using a computer keyboard is a very different experience from face to face communication. The type of information which might be readily disclosed online includes:

- name, age, gender, location;

- likes, dislikes, friends, enemies;

- worries, fears, hopes, dreams;

- plans;

- passwords, security codes;

- mistakes, embarrassments, family secrets;

- pictures, sound recordings, digital videos.

The groomer's objective is to gain power over the victim, and they may use the dialogue to help the victim to develop empathy, or a sense of trust for the groomer, possibly focussed on the particular vulnerabilities of the victim (see above). The groomer may seek to develop the dialogue so that the victim experiences pleasure from the communication, or at least from the associated sense of attention.

However, empathy may not play a significant role in all forms of internet grooming. The possibility of coercion increases as the victim shares more of their more intimate personal details with the groomer; some groomers have sent email attachments containing Trojan software to victims. The software, when run, allows the groomer to remotely control some functions of the victim's computer, which is frequently alarming for the victim. This type of activity might lead the prosecution to consider offences under the Computer Misuse Act 1990; files and programs stored on victim's computer may provide vital evidence in any future prosecution.

10.5.5 Suggestion and commitment

The groomer continues the communication but, for the first time, suggests or requests that the victim takes some specific action, such as communicating by telephone, meeting up or appearing on a webcam. The suggestion alone might constitute evidence of an offence under the Sexual Offences Act 2003:

- causing or inciting a child to engage in sexual activity (s 10);
- causing a child to watch a sexual act (s 12);
- arranging or facilitating commission of a child sex offence (s 14).

Again, any evidence of internet communications between the groomer and victim might be important in establishing that an offence has taken place.

The victim might reach the point of committing to some future action. The groomer may at this stage begin to deconstruct their cyber identity; for example, disclosing their true age, usually older than the victim had been led to believe. It is unclear whether this type of deconstruction is by necessity, (for instance if the groomer and victim are to meet and the groomer recognises that some aspects of their cyber personality are untenable face to face), or whether the groomer gains psychological satisfaction by divulging more of their true identity to their victim.

10.5.6 Discovery

It is obviously not always the case that internet grooming will be discovered. The groomer may turn elsewhere or the victim may not actually report the grooming to any other person or law enforcement authority. However, crimes of this type might be uncovered as a result of:

- Disclosure by the victim to a family member or friend;
- The offence being observed by a third party;
- Evidence that an offence has taken place coming to light;
- The offender confessing to the offence.

What is important is what happens next. It is not necessarily the case that the discovery of a crime of this kind will automatically lead to investigation and prosecution.

10.5.7 Suppression

Because of the personal and private nature of these offences, and fear of the possible consequences of disclosure, many such crimes go unreported. As was discussed earlier, paedophile crimes committed by priests during the 1940s have taken 60 years to resolve because of suppression and fear. It is now widely understood that many such crimes take place within families. Even if discovered, the possibility of disgrace and loss of social standing lead to hiding the failings of family members. The danger of suppressing crimes of this nature is obviously the fear of repetition, in addition to the loss of justice for the victims. If paedophiles consider themselves to be invulnerable to prosecution, there are seemingly no barriers to repeat offences being committed.

10.5.8 Prosecution

An offence is committed under s 15 of the Sexual Offences Act 2003 if it can be demonstrated that, as a result of internet grooming, a person meets with (or is travelling to meet) a victim. In the UK the sentence for any offence resulting from internet grooming is imprisonment for up to 10 years.

Questions

Robin Bryant & Sarah Bryant

1. How are digital technologies impacting on the 'traditional' models of paedophile activity and development?

2. Do we need to better distinguish between different forms of paedophile activity in terms of the potential future risk to children? For example, what are the links between utilising child pornography and the sexual abuse of children?

3. What were the key features of 'Operation Ore'?

4. Why is it an advantage for investigators to have some insight into the possible motivations of offenders involved in child pornography?

5. What are the aims of the VGT, and what steps have been taken to further these aims?

6. How might 'Web 2.0' affect the incidence of online grooming?

7. What offences may be committed as part of an online grooming process?

References

BBC (2001) Wickedness of Wonderland. BBC News [Online]. Available at: http://news.bbc.co.uk/1/hi/uk/1167879.stm (Accessed: Jul 1 2007).

BBC (2003) Online dragnet to thwart paedophiles. BBC News [Online]. Available at: http://news.bbc.co.uk/1/hi/technology/3330929.stm (Accessed: Jul 1 2007).

BBC (2007) LA Cardinal offers abuse apology. BBC News [Online]. Available at: http://news.bbc.co.uk/1/hi/world/americas/6900129.stm (Accessed: Jul 1 2007).

Billboard (2006) Appeals court upholds Glitter conviction. [Online]. Available at: http://billboard.com/bbcom/news/article_display.jsp?vnu_content_id=1002688981, (Accessed: Jul 1 2007).

Blogger (2007) Blogger. [Online]. Available at: https://www.blogger.com/start (Accessed: Jul 1 2007).

CEOP (2007) Child Exploitation and Online Protection Centre. [Online]. Available at: http://www.ceop.gov.uk/ (Accessed: Jul 1 2007).

CERN (1989) Information management: a proposal. [Online]. Available at: http://www.w3.org/History/1989/proposal.html (Accessed: Jul 1 2007).

Coffman, K.G. and Odlyzko, A.M. (2001) Growth of the internet. [Online]. Available at: http://www.dtc.umn.edu/~odlyzko/doc/oft.internet.growth.pdf (Accessed: Oct 10 2007).

Del.icio.us (2007) Del.icio.us social bookmarking. [Online]. Available at: http://del.icio.us/ (Accessed: Oct 10 2007).

Fickr (2007) Flickr. [Online]. Available at: http://flickr.com/ (Accessed: Jul 1 2007).

Hauben, M. (2007) The history of the ARPANET. [Online]. Available at: http://www.dei.isep.ipp.pt/~acc/docs/arpa.html (Accessed: Jul 1 2007).

MySpace (2007) UK MySpace A space for friends. [Online]. Available at: http://myspace.com/ (Accessed: Jul 1 2007).

O'Reilly Associates (2007) Controversy about our 'Web 2.0' service mark. [Online]. Available at: http://radar.oreilly.com/archives/2006/05/controversy_about_our_web_20_s.html (Accessed: Jul 1 2007).

Qi, M. and Edgar-Nevill, D. (2007) Tracking email offenders. ETHICOMP Working Conference 2007, Kunming, China, Apr 2–3, 2007.

Sheriff, L. (2007) Operation Ore: evidence of massive credit card fraud. [Online]. Available at: http://www.theregister.co.uk/2007/04/19/operation_ore_fraud/print.html (Accessed: Jul 1 2007).

USA Today (2007) Catholic Church settles sex-abuse allegations for $660M. [Online]. Available at: http://blogs.usatoday.com/ondeadline/2007/07/catholic-church.html (Accessed: Jul 1 2007).

VGT (2007) Virtual Global Taskforce. [Online]. Available at: http://www.virtualglobaltaskforce.com/index.asp (Accessed: Jul 1 2007).

Wiki (2007) Wiki.com. [Online]. Available at: http://wiki.com/ (Accessed: Jul 1 2007).

YouTube (2007) YouTube broadcast yourself. [Online]. Available at: http://youtube.com/ (Accessed: Jul 1 2007).

11
Digitalisation and Crime

Robin Bryant and Paul Stephens

When discussing digital crime, familiar examples are often proffered, such as cybercrime or computer hacking. There are however, examples of crimes in which the digital aspect (the 'digitalisation') has been a less obvious but nonetheless critical factor in the development and commissioning of a particular activity. In this chapter we examine mobile phones, games consoles, money laundering and the provision of pharmaceutical drugs as four such examples. In each case we offer some comment on the digital nature of these crimes.

Writing in 1998, David Wall outlined the four broad ways in which the internet in particular has impacted on crime, through:

- cyber-trespass (hacking which ranges from ethical hacking to information warfare);

- cyber-thefts (fraud, appropriation of intellectual property);

- cyber-obscenities (pornography, sex-trade);

- cyber-violence (stalking, hate-speech) (Wall, 1998).

Although the internet has certainly played a role in money laundering, and in crimes involving mobile phones, games consoles, and the provision of

Investigating Digital Crime   Edited by Robin Bryant and Sarah Bryant
© 2008 John Wiley & Sons, Ltd

pharmaceutical drugs, none of the crimes fit neatly into just one of Wall's four categories. In some cases they instead straddle the categories or possess features which seem not to fall under any particular heading. Rather, the crimes considered in this chapter are examples of how digitalisation (see Chapter 1) of information, technology and communication is having a wider affect on patterns of behaviour, not only in terms of organised crime but also in terms of involving otherwise law-abiding people.

11.1 Mobile phones

In the West the mobile phone is now ubiquitous, and indeed in some countries market penetration exceeds 100 per cent; in Italy there are 12 mobile phones in active use for every 10 people in the population (Ofcom, 2006). Until the early 1990s, mobile phones were too expensive and impractical for everyday use, and employed analogue systems to communicate (see section 1.2 in Chapter 1). However, two developments led to a rapid take up of mobile phone use: the advent of a cellular and digital system (which subsequently allowed 'roaming' both locally and internationally using GSM) and new payment arrangements, such as reductions in cost and the phasing of costs, including the use of pre-paid mobiles. The market price of many makes of mobile phones has also fallen, due to mass production and miniaturisation, although a parallel increase in functionality has created a wider price gap than in the past between makes and models of mobiles.

In the pre-digital era of mobile phones, information about a phone (such as its serial number) and the calls themselves were sent unencrypted over the network. Therefore, it was relatively easy for a motivated individual to eavesdrop on a network and obtain information about a phone. Serial numbers were then used to illegally clone mobile phones which could then be used to make calls at the expense of a legitimate subscriber.

More recently in the UK the digital nature of mobile phones has been exploited in a similar type of crime. The process involves reprogramming a phone's unique international mobile equipment identity (IMEI) number, and is known as 'unblocking' – not to be confused with the legal activity of 'unlocking'. The IMIE number is normally 14 or 15 digits in length and is usually printed somewhere on the phone, often under the battery. Alternatively, it can be accessed on most phones by entering the key sequence *#06#). Note that the IMEI number of a phone does not change with a change of SIM card – the IMEI number is stored within the memory of the phone itself and therefore identifies the phone, and not the subscriber who owns or uses the phone. (Information concerning the subscriber is usually stored on the SIM card.)

The IMEI number is transmitted whenever the phone tries to access a network and periodically when requested by the service operator; these processes are invisible to the user. The transmitted IMEI number is checked against a central Equipment Identity Register (EIR), the UKSEIR within the UK. There are three possible outcomes:

- The IMEI number is 'white-listed' and the phone is allowed to be connected to the network.

- The IMEI number is 'grey-listed' which means it is under observation, although calls are still permitted.

- The IMEI number is 'black-listed', which means that the phone has been re-ported stolen, or access to the network is refused for some other reason; the phone is blocked.

The EIR is shared between all the major cellular networks, so a blocked stolen mobile phone (even with a valid SIM card) should remain blocked, at least in the UK. However, there is one obvious way around this; unblock a phone by changing its IMEI number. This is illegal, as is the offer to change an IMEI number, an offence under the Mobile Telephones (Re-Programming) Act 2002, (with subsequent additions through the Violent Crime Reduction Act 2006).

However, information on how to re-program an IMEI number was widely available through the internet in the late 1990s and early part of this century, as were duplicate IMEI numbers that were known to work. In one case (the BT cellnet network, now O_2) a duplicate number was used more than 9000 times before being blocked (John Denham in a parliamentary debate; HC Deb 22 July 2002 c709). In 2002 it was estimated that the IMEI number had been changed in 75 per cent of stolen phones (HC Deb 22 July 2002 c709). Companies such as Nokia have attempted to counter the illegal unblocking of their mobile

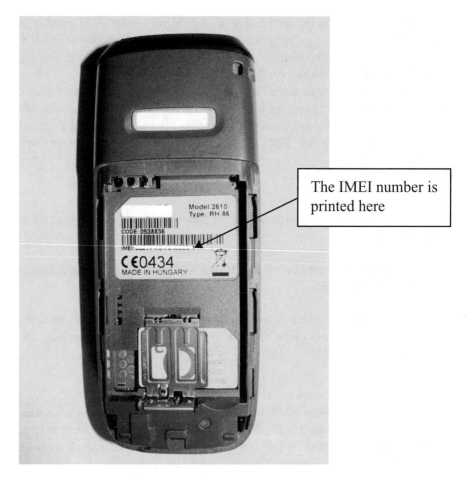

The IMEI number is printed here

Figure 11.1   The position of the IMEI number

phones by writing the IMEI number to a new read-only part of the mobile's memory.

The digital nature of this crime is evident through three main characteristics. First, the exploitation of the digital nature of the IMEI information storage, and an understanding of the algorithm used to check the possible authenticity of an IMEI number was an important precursor to any form of subsequent criminal activity. Secondly, both the hardware and software 'solutions' to changing an IMEI number relied upon both this understanding and the digital nature of the phones themselves. The hardware involved, often called a 'chipping kit' was available for approximately £50 (Ward, 2002). Finally, both the information and the associated software were distributed through the internet. It is very unlikely, if only for pragmatic reasons, that this software could have been distributed in any other way, given its use for illegal activities.

Mobile Phone Forensics

Robin Bryant

Mobile phones often feature within crime; they may be used as the means for relatively anonymous communication between conspirators (often using prepaid accounts). The digitalisation of mobile phones has provided new opportunities for investigators; valuable information (both intelligence and evidence) may be obtained from mobile phones. This has given rise to the developing field of 'mobile phone forensics' which comprises two interrelated activities:

- analysis of the phone itself; and

- analysis of the associated network traffic and information (for example, the location of a mobile station – the combination of a mobile phone and its SIM card – using cell site use and coverage density maps).

A mobile phone will often store apparently deleted information (as will many devices with electronic memory) and many users appear to be completely unaware of this. Text messages are stored either on the SIM card or within the integral memory of the mobile phone itself (or both). In most cases at least some of the deleted text messages still resident on the SIM card can be recovered (somewhat less so in the case of the mobile phone memory) using forensically validated techniques. The figure below is an example of deleted text messages recovered from a mobile phone using 'USIM Detective' commercial software (Quantaq Solutions, 2007). Note that there is no guarantee that the text message may not have been subsequently altered by a suspect after it was first received.

Section 9 - Deleted text messages

Record	Status	Message	Origin	SMSC
5	Message received. Timestamp: 20 Mar 2007 09:10:41 GMT, read status unknown	Think I just saw Emily but not sure. Would she be walking up Waterloo Road at 9am?	+447974821234 (Gary)	+447973100983
6	Message received. Timestamp: 24 Mar 2007 16:01:20 GMT, read status unknown	HT 1:1. Coasting then Chart sent off, Smith just stopped from walking off after attacking Chart. Possible racist incident	+447974821234 (Gary)	+447973100983
7	Message received. Timestamp: 24 Mar 2007 16:55:18 GMT, read status unknown	2:1 Dover FT	+447974821234 (Gary)	+447973100983
9	Message received. Timestamp: 28 Mar 2007 12:59:08 GMT+1, read status unknown	O2: Thanks for your request. Your Euro Bolt On will be available within 48hrs. Pls have £1.99 on yr balance until you get our confirmation text. Terms@o2.co.uk	"O2/UK@"	+447802000332
10	Message received. Timestamp: 29 Mar 2007 09:04:19 GMT+1, read status unknown	Your request for EURO has not been successful as your tariff is ineligible.Please call Customer Service for info on upgrading your tariff on 08705678678	"O2-UK@"	+447802000332
11	Message received. Timestamp: 31 Mar 2007 16:51:48 GMT+1, read status unknown	FT 5-0, walker 2,dryden 2,humphreys.wallis good.peter.	+447835734321 (Peter)	+447802000332
12	Message received. Timestamp: 31 Mar 2007 16:52:41 GMT+1, read status unknown	And river end first half!strange.	+447835734321 (Peter)	+447802000332
13	Message received. Timestamp: 5 Apr 2007 11:32:59 GMT+1, read status unknown	O2 Roaming: With your O2 mobile you need to include +33 to call within France, and do not need +44 to call the UK. For voicemail dial 901.	"Roaming@"	+447802000332
14	Message received. Timestamp: 24 Oct 2004 09:35:52 GMT+1, read status unknown	Okay the frequencys to try 6195, 12095, 9410, 15485, 7320 these are all the ones listed under europe	+447754941299	+447802092035
15	Message received. Timestamp: 11 Apr 2007 05:13:23 GMT+1, read status unknown	Hi Rik, Small world - am in Dubai and two colleagues from work here. Both very good. See soon, Bill Brown	+447917013304 (Bill Brown)	+447785016005
16	Message received. Timestamp: 13 Apr 2007 09:28:16 GMT+1, read status unknown	Hey mummy. Are u going 2 want supper 2nite? What time u arive about? X	+447716851212 (Jenny)	+447802000332
17	Message received. Timestamp: 18 Apr 2007 08:50:43 GMT+1, read status unknown	Happy birthday:])	+447974821234 (Gary)	+447973074999

Figure 11.2   Recovered deleted SMS text messages from a mobile phone SIM card

Reference

Quantaq Solutions (2007) *USIM detective* Available at: http://www.quantaq.com/
    usimdetective.htm. [Online]. (Accessed: Oct 18 2007).

11.2 Games consoles

Many readers will be familiar with the current crop of popular games consoles, such as Nintendo's Wii, Microsoft's Xbox 360 and Sony's PlayStation 3. The first widely available consoles (such as the Nintendo Entertainment System, or NES) appeared in UK homes in the early to mid 1980s. Modern day games consoles vary in capability, function and cost, however they all share common features. Most modern games consoles have both hardware (the console itself, containing microprocessors and memory) and software (usually in the form of a disc, cartridge or some other form of proprietary format). Much of the architecture of these machines is similar to the PC; some consoles are also capable of playing audio CDs and DVDs.

Without the associated games software, games consoles are of limited interest to potential purchasers. Therefore, consumers need to acquire the games, frequently from the manufacturer of the console, though other companies may also be licensed to produce games (software) for particular consoles. Designers, manufacturers and producers all have a serious interest in protecting the intellectual property rights of their products, primarily in terms of preventing illegal copying.

Manufacturers may also place restrictions on the distribution rights of games media (for example, for the PlayStation 2 and Xbox) whereby games available in one country or region are not permitted to be used (they will not work unmodified) on a console designed for, and distributed in, a second country or region. For example, the Xbox console (the predecessor of the current Xbox 360) as sold in the UK will not play games sold in the US market, nor will it (in its commercially available form) play illegal or 'backup' copies.

However, for a number of reasons (for example, availability and cost) some users of the Xbox have attempted to circumvent this hardware protection by modifying ('modding') an Xbox, or by purchasing a modified console. The particular modification, often called 'chipping', involves replacing the genuine BIOS chip of an Xbox with a modified chip. This removes the region coding protection, so copies of games from other regions can be used, but more significantly (for the average gamer in the UK), copies of games will also play, and these illegal copies are usually much cheaper than the original and authorised versions. Similar modification systems have been devised for the Nintendo Game Cube, the Sony Playstation 2 and the recent Nintendo DS. Unsurprisingly, chipping is illegal in the UK under an EU copyright directive, and there have been a number of prosecutions (BBC, 2005)

When Microsoft designed the successor to its Xbox console (the Xbox 360) the piracy problems encountered with the original were certainly taken into account. Microsoft claimed that they had:

> made improvements on both the hardware and software side to protect Xbox 360 against piracy and modding. With Xbox 360, we had the benefit of learning from our experiences on Xbox. This allowed us to identify points of weakness that were exploited by hackers in the first generation and to eliminate those vulnerabilities in Xbox 360 (cited by Evers, 2005).

Despite this, rumours still circulate about the existence of modding code that will 'flash' the Xbox 360 firmware and allow the use of illegally copied games.

The digital aspects of this particular crime feature in two main respects. Firstly, there was the 'dumping' of the original BIOS of the Xbox (perhaps made possible because of lax security; see Steil, 2005), which provided access to significant information, facilitating the development of modified consoles which could play illegal and other region copies of games. Whereas in the past, highly technical information of this kind would have been restricted to a few knowledgeable and talented enthusiasts, the advent of the internet provided a means for both the rapid dissemination of information and for discussions leading to the development of new techniques. It is unlikely, for example, that details would have been published by a popular games magazine (some of which are linked to manufacturers as the 'official' games magazine for that particular console), or broadcast on a technology programme or gaming show on television.

Second, commercial entrepreneurs working in this legally 'grey' area can exploit 'hobbyist' knowledge and produce devices which require very little knowledge or skill on the part of prospective purchasers, giving rise to a small and presumably sufficiently profitable industry (see for example modchipworld.co.uk).

11.3 Money laundering

Money laundering is the process by which illegally gained income (for example, through trafficking in drugs or running a brothel) is made to look legitimate. That is, the 'dirty' money is washed to make it appear 'clean'. (The origins of the term are often assigned, probably erroneously, to the activities of the notorious 1930s gangster Al Capone and his Laundromat business, which was used to disguise criminal proceeds. Instead it is thought that the term is more likely to have been first used during the 'Watergate' scandal in the 1970s).

Money laundering predates the digital era. Indeed, criminal activity has long been associated with the generation of large amounts of cash, on occasions so large as to prove problematic for the criminals concerned. Although it might appear that cash is an infinitely elastic and flexible commodity, it soon becomes apparent to even a moderately successful criminal that its use is severely limited. In the past, popular accounts of organised criminals would often describe how illegally gained cash was laundered through purchase of cars, houses and pubs, which then appeared to be legitimately owned. However these avenues have been steadily closed for the criminals involved; above certain limits (which reflect the money laundering regulations now in existence in many countries) cash will not be accepted for property, investments, goods or services, and any attempt to directly circumvent these restrictions is likely to lead to suspicion and even a report to

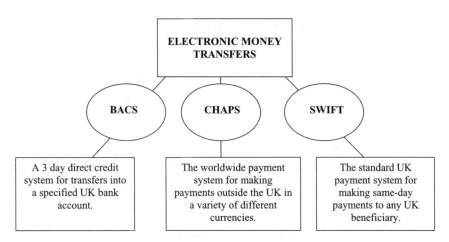

Figure 11.3 Electronic money transfer methods

the appropriate authorities. SWIFT is controlled particularly tightly, rendering it unattractive to money launderers.

In the UK, a 'Suspicious Activity Report' may be made to SOCA, the Serious Organised Crime Agency. The data shown in figure 11.4 shows the value of the illegal drugs trade globally (UNODC, 2006), most of which is cash or cash equivalents.

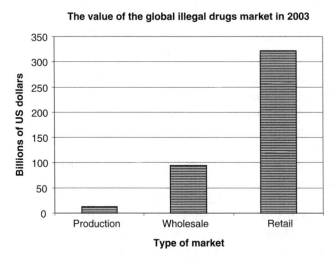

Figure 11.4 The value of the illegal drugs market

11.3.1 The money laundering process

A common way of conceptualising money laundering (e.g. FAFT, 2007) is to posit the existence of three distinct, but nonetheless interrelated, stages; placement, layering and integration. However, not all money laundering activities will involve all these stages, and some also include further stages. The flowchart in Figure 11.5 shows the key aspects of the process, and some common examples of how each stage may be achieved.

Digital cash and internet communication may now be involved in all three of the 'classic' stages of money laundering. As an example, consider a traditional form of placement in the UK; a winning betting slip is purchased for a sum higher than its face value. (For example, a £10 bet on a horse with odds 25 to one should be worth £260 but may be purchased by a small scale money launderer for £300.) The advantage for the launderer here is that the betting slip ostensibly provides an apparently legitimate means of having obtained the cash, concealing its true origins. In practice, this form of money laundering is quite limited in scale and relatively easy to detect if repeated enough times. In the digital era however, a similar technique involving online (or 'remote') gambling is not as restricted in scope, and is more difficult to detect. As Renade *et al.* note

> As a by-product of the evolution of remote gambling, there appears to be
> a money laundering 'arms race' in operation, with criminals exploiting
> loopholes or weaknesses in the system and governments and operators
> working to plug those gaps and strengthen those weaknesses (Renade
> *et. al.*, 2006, p. 21).

There are several reasons for this. First, there is very little control of online gambling; some online casinos in particular do not always exercise the usual 'due diligence' procedures normally associated with terrestrial gambling. (However, casinos operating from UK premises are treated in a similar way to UK financial institutions as far as money laundering regulations are concerned.) Second, online gambling would appear to offer greater scope for the electronic smurfing of larger amounts into smaller amounts, particularly given the large number of games being played online and their 24-hour nature. This is because of the possibility of automated electronic smurfing (similar in method to the legitimate use of automated bidding software used with online auction houses). Finally, this form of gambling lacks any form of human contact, and getting to know the customer is an important factor in traditional money laundering prevention. Perhaps

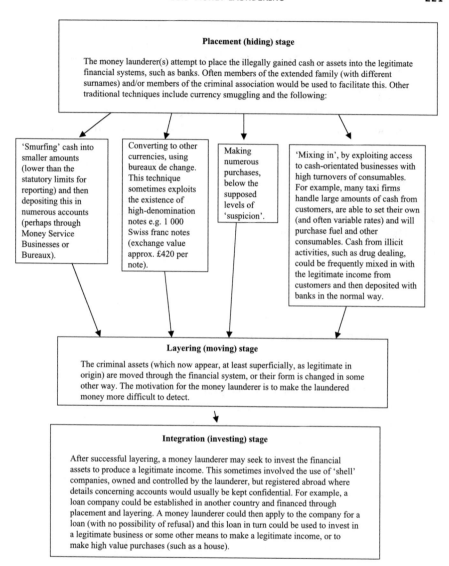

Figure 11.5 Key stages in money laundering

inevitably, money laundering through online casinos has been given the moniker of 'cyberlaundering'.

In the past, the various stages of money laundering would almost certainly have left a paper trail, but now almost every stage can potentially be conducted electronically, in a digital format. Given the large amount of financial electronic traffic, by no means all transactions will be permanently recorded and this fact may well be exploited by money launderers (FAFT, 2004, p. 4). This ephemeracy, (in addition to the speed of transactions and the placement and layering options made available through the internet) undoubtedly facilitates and stimulates the development of new forms of money laundering

For example, with the development of 'e-money', entirely digital forms of cash are now possible. E-money may be either hardware or software based and involves the prepay 'charging up' of a card or electronic account. The e-money may then be used in similar ways to traditional cash, and indeed some forms of e-money are referred to as 'electronic purchases'. At the time of writing, there is very little control over e-money systems, creating an attendant risk of money laundering, at least for relatively small amounts of cash (JMLSG, 2007). In the UK, a consultation is underway to consider whether the identity details of an e-money purchaser (for transactions above certain limits) should be requested and recorded.

11.4 Pharmaceutical drugs

In the UK the prescription and supply of pharmaceutical drugs (often medicines used to prevent or treat illness and/or its symptoms) are strictly controlled. Selling these drugs without the proper authority is an offence under UK law, punishable by fine and/or imprisonment. For example, section 8 (3) (a) of the Medicines Act 1968 makes it an offence to sell, or offer to sell, a medicinal product, except than in accordance with a wholesale dealer's licence. If the pharmaceutical drugs are fakes but carry recognised trade names such as 'Viagra' then prosecution is also possible under the Trade Marks Act 1994 and the Criminal Law Act 1977. Various other pieces of legislation may also be relevant (e.g. the Medicines (Advertising) Regulations 1994).

Under the Medicines Act 1968, there are three types of pharmaceutical drugs:

- general sales list ('GSL') medicines (such as paracetamol) which may be sold from a wide range of outlets including shops and supermarkets;

- pharmacy medicines ('P') , which may only be sold from pharmacies (under the supervision of the pharmacist) but do not necessarily require a prescription from a GP or similar health professional (such as 'morning after' pills);

- prescription-only medicines ('POM'), which also can only be sold from pharmacies but do require a prescription from a GP or similar (such as 'antibiotics').

Up until the mid 19th century, the dispensing of medicines was largely unregulated and anyone could term themselves a 'chemist' or 'druggist'. Under the 1868 Pharmacy Act a register was established, listing people who were qualified to dispense 'poisons' (which included opiates), but it was not until the early part of the 20th century that the dispensing of medicines became comprehensively regulated (Smith, 2004, p.43). Throughout the remainder of the 20th century, responsibility for prescribing and dispensing prescription-only medicines lay firmly with the professions involved.

However, until the advent of the NHS in 1948 the availability of GP prescription-only medicine was patchy and (other than in the most life-threatening cases) largely unavailable for economic reasons to many ordinary citizens, particularly women. Instead, people used cheap 'self-help' medicines widely available without prescription from high street chemists. There is therefore only a short history in the UK (of 60 years or so) of relatively cheap and wide access to officially prescribed and effective medicines available through professional agencies, and a much longer history of taking recourse to local chemist remedies and 'patent' off the shelf medicines.

We now have a move in the UK towards 'patient empowerment' with the creation of 'patient experts' who use websites to discover more about their conditions or even to check diagnoses (Fox *et al.*, 2004). Coinciding with this, particularly since the mid 1980s, there has been an increasing tendency (Bond, 2001) to 'deregulate' selected medicines from prescription-only to pharmacy medicines; that is from POM to P (and perhaps then to GSL). An example is hydrocortisone cream, an anti-inflammatory used to treat the symptoms of various skin problems.

Patients may also have doubts about the suitability and range of treatments available from the NHS, and this possibility has attracted significant attention from the media. The availability of some medicines is often perceived to vary depending on where a patient lives in the UK (the so-called 'postcode lottery'), although these forms of 'rationing' only apply to a very small number of drugs. (There was a particular controversy concerning the availability of Herceptin, a treatment for some forms of breast cancer, which received widespread publicity).

Online web-based pharmacies began to appear in 1999 (reported by the National Center on Addiction and Substance Abuse, (CASA, 2007)), advertising POM medicines for sale, as well as GSL medicines. Examples of pharmaceutical drugs available over the internet include those usually prescribed to treat erectile dysfunction, and appetite suppressants to assist weight loss, but many others are available for a wide range of conditions (Wilkinson, 2007). In February 2006, one researcher counted a total of 344 websites as either advertising or selling controlled pharmaceutical drugs (Wilkinson, 2007). By the following year, the number had increased to approximately 580, only two of which were 'officially licensed' (CASA, 2007).

Of course, for all purchases made on line there is the obvious danger of becoming the victim of fraud or deception; that is paying for goods but not receiving them, and for drugs it is particularly difficult to judge the quality of the product received. Some fake drugs contain little more than powdered chalk, whilst others only contain a tiny amount of the active ingredient. However, medical professionals and others have identified a number of potential problems. The patient may purchase a drug that is inappropriate as a consequence of an incorrect self diagnosis, possibly through completing online questionnaires offered by some online pharmacies. Even if the patient has correctly diagnosed the disorder, the drug or the standard dosage may not be appropriate for that particular person due to:

- his or her age or sex;
- other medical conditions and general state of health;
- interactions with other drugs he or she may be taking.

If the dosage taken is too high, excessive side effects may be experienced, some of which might be dangerous, and of course, too low a dosage is likely to be ineffective. In addition, the self-medicator may not be able to:

- recognise side effects;
- monitor any beneficial effects;
- recognise that the drug is unsuitable for other reasons.

Many POM drugs available today have far more powerful effects than traditional GSL medicines, and should also be noted that pharmacy and medical training courses take several years.

It would appear that the UK authorities can only currently take direct action against non-licensed online pharmacies that are registered in the UK (MHRA, 2007). However, the IP addresses of many internet pharmacies are actually located abroad even though they may superficially appear to be UK based. For example, the website 'Online Pharmacy UK' offers 'prescription medicine on line at discount pharmacy prices ... with no prescription' (On Line Pharmacy UK, 2007). A WHOIS lookup on the domain name in September 2007 showed that the registrant's address was given as 'South Shields, Florida' and the IP address was located in San Diego in California.

Despite these potential problems, the internet supply of pharmaceutical drugs may be attractive to some consumers for the following reasons:

- limited access to medicines in some countries (INCB, 2007);

- the high cost of medicines in some countries;

- convenience; ordering online and home delivery may be particularly important for those encountering problems with mobility;

- privacy; as the INCB (2007, p. 3) note

> The ability to obtain controlled drugs through the internet offers a degree of privacy, as there are no medical records indicating that the person has been taking a course of treatment for an ailment or illness, which might pose problems regarding that person's current or prospective employment or health insurance.

Further, the existence and efficacy of some prescription drugs like Viagra is widely known, but seeking treatment for erectile dysfunction may be a source of embarrassment and online pharmacies may appear to offer a confidential solution;

- a drug may not be licensed for use in the UK but trials elsewhere suggest it may be effective. As Fox et al. note (2004, p.1301), the internet in particular 'provides new opportunities both for publishing information about diseases and to enable patients and others to discuss conditions collaboratively' often in online forums. These discussions often include news about promising trials and this in turn may generate a demand for drugs from online pharmacies;

- to deliberately circumvent the official mechanisms. This might be the case with performance-enhancing drugs and steroids, as well as weight-loss drugs.

Some online pharmacies may see themselves as offering a genuine service, perhaps for some of the reasons listed above, and endeavour to supply genuine medicines and offer sound advice. The Royal Pharmaceutical Society of Great Britain is piloting the use of a logo to indicate bona fide online pharmacies in attempt to distinguish them from those that may pose dangers to the public.

Regulatory body actions against online pharmacies

The Medicines and Healthcare products Regulatory Agency (the MHRA) is an executive agency within the Department Of Health and is the regulatory body that carries most of the responsibility for investigating illegal UK-based online pharmacies. The MHRA employs its own investigators as part of their 'Enforcement and Intelligence Group', numbering about 40 officers (Ahmed & Deets, 2006).

Investigators are now able to access communications data (including itemised call records, routing information and subscriber details) held by communication service providers (e.g. ISPs) as part of their investigations. Statutory Instrument SI 2003, No. 3172 of the Regulation of Investigatory Powers Act 2000 provides MHRA officers of a certain seniority (or above) with the powers to 'acquire' communications data falling within sections 21(4) (b) and (c) of the Act.

'Operation Stormgrand'

In 2002, customs officials at Stansted airport intercepted a parcel containing fake Viagra tablets, addressed to a man in Leicestershire. This was followed by further seizures at Stansted and another airport. The subsequent investigation by the MHRA uncovered a major conspiracy involving the smuggling of POMs (counterfeit and genuine) into the UK. The counterfeit drugs included fake Viagra, Cialis and Propecia. They were sourced from China and Pakistan and in some cases contained up to 90% of the genuine article. The non-counterfeit POMs were Sildenafil, Citrate and Tadalafil.

Prior to 2005 (when arrests were made), the counterfeit drugs were used to supply websites and spammers illegally offering POMs for sale. The criminal operation involved 'fake packaging, labels, patient information leaflets and even fraudulent documents laying false trails to bona fide companies' (Boseley, 2007). In 2004 genuine Cialis was temporarily withdrawn from circulation as it was felt that the high proportion of counterfeit Cialis in circulation could potentially undermine the position of the regulated and genuine drug.

In September 2007, four men were convicted on a number of counts, including conspiracy to 'evade the prohibition on the unauthorised use of a trade mark in relation to goods', contrary to section 92(1) of the Trade Marks Act 1994 and section 1(1) of the Criminal Law Act 1977 (MRHA, 2007).

'Operation Rome'

In September 2006, enforcement officers from the MHRA, accompanied by police officers from a number of UK forces, carried out an operation against premises in Essex, Middlesex, Kent and Lancashire connected with five internet online pharmacy sites (MHRA, 2006). The MHRA officers seized Kamagra (an unlicensed medicine to treat male impotence) and Ephedrine (a POM, frequently used unofficially as a stimulant and appetite suppressant).

References

Ahmed, N. & Deets, M. (2006) *Medicines and Healthcare products Regulatory Agency (MHRA) Enforcement Group and its UK Medicines Anti-counterfeiting Strategy.* [Online] Available at: http://www.touchbriefings.com/pdf/2404/ACF1C8.pdf. (Accessed: Oct 15 2007).

Boseley, S. (2007) *Made for 25p, sold for £15. The fake Viagra that netted pill gang millions.* Guardian Unlimited [Online]. Available at: http://www.guardian.co.uk/medicine/story/0,,2171477,00.html#article_continue (Accessed: Oct 17 2007).

MHRA (2006) *Press release: Medicines investigators tackle the illegal sale of medicines over the internet.*[Online]. Available at: http://www.mhra.gov.uk/home/idcplg?IdcService=GET_FILE&dDocName=CON2024823&RevisionSelectionMethod=LatestReleased (Accessed: Oct 15 2007).

MHRA (2007) *Press release: Counterfeit medicines gang convicted in Operation Stormgrand.* [Online]. Available at: http://www.mhra.gov.uk/home/idcplg?IdcService=GET_FILE&dDocName=CON2032386&RevisionSelectionMethod=LatestReleased. (Accessed: Oct 15 2007).

Those wishing to illegally sell pharmaceutical drugs on the internet are able to exploit a number of the common characteristics of the digitalisation of crime beyond those normally associated with cybercrime. First, (as with phishing) it is relatively easy to gain access to the digitalised versions of logos and trademarks of both pharmaceutical companies and their products. Sophisticated fraudsters will even examine the source code of a webpage to discover the types of font used by the companies in order to copy this and instil some kind of (probably subconscious) added confidence within the potential victim. Second, many pharmaceutical companies and health advice sites publish online detailed information concerning indications, cautions, contra-indications, side effects and dose. Until relatively recently this kind of information was only available through paper-based professional publications such as the *British National Formulary* (a joint publication of the British Medical Association and the Royal Pharmaceutical Society of Great Britain). The online information is easily adaptable for use in illegal sales of pharmaceutical drugs.

Questions

Robin Bryant & Sarah Bryant

1. What is the difference between unblocking and unlocking a mobile phone?

2. What sort of information may be obtained from a mobile phone by a specialist investigator?

3. Why might a gamer prefer to have a 'modded' games console rather than a standard console?

4. How has the internet contributed to fraud associated with games consoles?

5. Which of the three 'classic' stages of money laundering are likely to be most affected by the growth of digital technologies?

6. What sorts of offences may be associated with online gambling?

7. Why is it an offence to sell certain categories of pharmaceutical drugs online?

8. What are some reasons why a person may prefer to obtain drugs online rather than from their local pharmacy?

References

BBC (2005) Man convicted for chipping Xbox. BBC News. [Online]. Available at: http://news.bbc.co.uk/1/hi/technology/4650225.stm (Accessed: Oct 11 2007).

Bond, C. (2001) POM to P – implications for practice pharmacists. *Primary Care Pharmacy* **2** Mar 2001: pp. 5–7.

CASA (2007)   'You've Got Drugs!' IV: Prescription Drug Pushers on the Internet. [Online]. Available at: http://www.casacolumbia.org/absolutenm/articlefiles/380-YGD4%20Report.pdf (Accessed: Oct 10 2007).

Evers, J. (2005) Hackers find first Xbox 360 cracks. [Online]. Available at: http://www.news.com/Hackers-find-first-Xbox-360-cracks/2100–7349_3–5999169.html (Accessed: Oct 10 2007).

FAFT (2004) Report on Money Laundering Typologies. [Online]. Available at: http://www.oecd.org/dataoecd/19/11/33624379.PDF (Accessed: Oct 10 2007).

FAFT (2007) Money Laundering FAQ. [Online]. Available at: http://www.oecd.org/document/29/0,3343,en_32250379_32235720_33659613_1_1_1_1,00.html (Accessed: Oct 10 2007).

Fox, N., Ward, K. and O'Rourke, A. (2004) The 'expert patient': empowerment or medical dominance? The case of weight loss, pharmaceutical drugs and the Internet. *Social Science & Medicine* **60**:1299–1309.

INCB (2007) Report of the International Narcotics Control Board for 2006. [Online]. Available at: http://www.incb.org/incb/annual_report_2006.html (Accessed: Oct 10 2007).

JMSLG (2007) 3: Electronic money. [Online]. Available at: http://www.jmlsg.org.uk/bba/jsp/polopoly.jsp?d=763&a=10236 (Accessed: Oct 10 2007).

MRHA (2007) Buying medicines over the internet. [Online]. Available at: http://www.mhra.gov.uk/home/idcplg?IdcService=SS_GET_PAGE&nodeId=254 (Accessed: Oct 10 2007).

Ofcom (2006) Ofcom International Communications Market Report. [Online]. Available at: http://www.ofcom.org.uk/research/cm/icmr06/ (Accessed: Oct 11 2007).

On Line Pharmacy UK (2007) On Line Pharmacy UK. [Online]. Available at: http://www.on-linepharmacyuk.com/ (Accessed: Oct 10 2007)

Renade, S., Bailey, S. and Harvey A. (2006) A literature review and survey of statistical sources on remote gambling. [Online]. Available at: http://www.culture.gov.uk/NR/rdonlyres/E0A395C1–35CC-4717-BF00-B1F6BD3A6B76/0/RemoteGambling_RSeReport.pdf (Accessed: Oct 10 2007)

Smith, Dame Janet (2004) *Shipman Inquiry Fourth Report – The Regulation of Controlled Drugs in the Community.* Published 15 July 2004 Command Paper Cm 6249.

Steil, M. (2005) 17 mistakes Microsoft made in the Xbox security system. [Online]. Available at: http://events.ccc.de/congress/2005/fahrplan/attachments/591-paper_xbox.pdf (Accessed: Oct 11 2007).

UNODC (2006) World Drug Report. [Online]. Available at: http://www.unodc.org/unodc/en/world_drug_report.html (Accessed: Oct 10 2007).

Wall, D. (1998) Policing and the regulation of cyberspace. *Criminal Law Review special issue Crime, Criminal Justice and the Internet* (1998): pp. 79–91.

Ward (2002) How to hack your mobile phone. [Online]. Available at: http://news.bbc.co.uk/1/hi/sci/tech/1966381.stm (Accessed: 11 Oct 2007).

Wilkinson, L. (2007) Internet access to controlled prescription drugs. [Online]. Available at: http://www.drugpreventionevidence.info/web/Internet_access_to_controlled_prescription_drugs344.asp (Accessed: Oct 10 2007).

12

Criminological and Motivational Perspectives

Robin Bryant and Angus Marshall

As Newburn notes (2007, p.839), 'criminology and psychology have strong connections in their respective histories' and it is perhaps therefore inevitable that theoretical approaches to understanding digital crime tend to draw upon both criminological and psychological (particularly motivational) perspectives. In this chapter we examine a number of criminological and psychological theories and discuss their application to particular digital crimes. We conclude with a description of on-going research into 'cyberprofiling'.

12.1 Criminological perspectives

There has been some debate concerning whether criminology has kept pace with developments in digital crime. It is interesting to note, for example, that even the 2007 fourth edition of the influential *Oxford Handbook of Criminology* (a 'set book' on undergraduate courses in criminology in many UK universities) has no dedicated chapter or section on digital crime although it does devote sections of the Handbook to other specific forms of crime such 'violent crime' and 'drugs,

Investigating Digital Crime   Edited by Robin Bryant and Sarah Bryant
© 2008 John Wiley & Sons, Ltd

alcohol and crime' (Maguire *et al.*, 2007). Jaishankar (2007, p.1) goes as far to suggest that:

> criminology has been remiss in its research into the phenomena of cyber crime and has been slow to recognize the importance of cyberspace in changing the nature and scope of offending and victimization.

There are a number of possible responses to this criticism. Most of the criminological schools and theories pre-date the advent of digital crime. That is, they were never 'meant' to explain or theorise about online fraud or credit card cloning but were instead much more general theories concerned with variously human nature, social interaction, the organisation of society and so on. Often they reflected the particular discipline from which they were drawn, for example biology or psychology (Burke, 2005, p.1). It is also highly simplistic to consider these theories in isolation or indeed to consider them as monolithic entities in some kind of competition with each other. None-the-less it is instructive to revisit a few of the more popular criminological theories and reassess them in the light of recent changes in the forms of criminal activity. In this way we illuminate both the nature of digital crime itself and some possible approaches to preventing and detecting such crimes.

In very general terms, we can think of three main 'schools' of criminological theory established in the 18th and 19th centuries, and their modern-day derivatives (Table 12.1).

Note however, that this is a highly simplified account and ignores important themes in criminology such as conflict theory, left realism and feminist perspectives, which are beyond the scope of this chapter. Below we consider an example of each school, and how they might be applied to a number of examples of digital crimes.

Table 12.1 Criminological theories and modern examples

School of criminological theory	Modern examples
Classical and neo-classical	Rational choice theory, routine activity theory
Positivist	Biosocial and psychological theories, the Chicago school, social learning (differential association) theory
Sociological	Strain (anomie) theory, social control theory, labelling

12.1.1 Routine activity theory

Routine activity theory (RAT; also known as routine activities theory) was first developed by the criminologists Ron Clarke and Marcus Felson in the 1980s and 1990s (Clarke and Felson, 1993), although it has its roots in much earlier classical and neo-classical theories. In the original formulation of RAT, crime (and in particular acquisitive crime) was posited as a function of three variables ranging over space and time:

- the existence of a suitable target;

- the presence of a motivated offender; and

- the absence of a suitable guardian (which includes non-human guardians, such as alarm systems).

Crime at a certain location and time would be more or less likely according to how these variables combined. Interestingly, Felson (1998, cited in Burke (2005)), later added a fourth variable to the routine activities mix, namely the absence of an 'intimate handler', a person who would normally exercise some restraining control over the potential offender. Examples of an intimate handler include a parent or significant other. Sometimes by necessity, sitting and using a PC tends to be a solitary activity, and it is far less obvious to an intimate handler that a person may be engaged in an online form of criminal activity. (See the variable C_g described in section 12.3 below).

As an example of 'conventional' RAT, consider a public car park with a significant frequency of car stereo thefts. A number of the local residents from the adjacent housing estate are recidivist volume crime offenders, and the car park is poorly lit and largely unsupervised, and there are no CCTV cameras nearby. In terms of the RAT variables we have:

- suitable targets in the form of cars with valuables;
- motivated offenders from the neighbouring estate; and
- poor security and monitoring; there are few capable guardians.

A high level of crime at this particular car park therefore comes as no surprise to the RAT theorist.

RAT has been particularly influential in terms of approaches to crime reduction and is almost an orthodoxy in terms of 'official' ways of conceptualising high volume acquisitive crime (e.g. Home Office, 2006). Even in the digital era, RAT is also considered by some to be almost 'universally applicable' as a means of gaining insight into crime prevention (Farrell and Pease, 2006, p.180).

A RAT-based crime reduction strategy for the car park scenario above would involve an analysis of each of the three components described above. In terms of the existence of suitable targets and motivated offenders little could be done, at least in the short term. However, there are some reasonably obvious ways in which we could increase the guardianship, including installing CCTV or monitoring the car park in some other way.

However, now consider the illegal downloader of copyrighted music from the internet, probably using peer-to-peer software. This activity requires minimal technical knowledge on the part of the downloader, and there is no shortage of suitable targets. For example, a search using the popular BitTorrent site http://www.mininova.org/ in August 2007 for music by the late Johnny Cash gave 212 torrents (including one of 2.89 Gb in size, containing 47 albums by Cash, comprising almost all his artistic output).

The forms of motivation here are likely to include:

- relatively instant gratification;

- low financial cost (which is in any case difficult to disaggregate from the monthly broadband costs);

- a greater range of product 'on offer', including unauthorised or unissued recordings, foreign language albums and 'bootlegs'; and

- libertarian beliefs in the 'freedom' of intellectual property (Wall, 2007, p. 97).

At any time there are likely to be millions of people around the world using peer-to-peer software to share copyrighted music. For example, the popular BitTorrent client Amazeus (downloading BitTorrents requires both information about the torrent itself and a client to perform the uploading and downloading) regularly reports in excess of one million simultaneous users (though not all will be sharing copyrighted music). Although there are occasional highly publicised reports of filesharers (particularly uploaders) being pursued for costs by the music industry (e.g. BBC, 2005), relatively low-volume filesharers are likely to be aware that the probability of detection is small and the consequences (in the UK) normally involve paying costs, or facing civil action rather than criminal proceedings. There is the distinct lack of any sense of a capable guardian.

| Search in category: | All | Anime | Books | Games | Movies | Music | Pictures | Software | TV Shows | Other | | | |

Added	Name		Size	Seeds	Leechers
24 Jul 07	Johnny Cash - An American Icon - 2 DVD's + 2 CD's Boxset		5.91 GB	11	66
29 Nov 06	Johnny Cash Live at Montrelux 1994		3.81 GB	1	3
07 Jul 07	Johnny Cash Shows 3-24 & 3-31, 1971		2.96 GB	10	2
29 Aug 07	Johnny Cash Huge Collection (47 albums) [zgbTrnt]-(Demonoid com) 1192170 7602		2.89 GB	31	154
18 Sep 06	Johnny Cash: Complete Recording Sessions: 1954-1969		2.55 GB	13	10
30 Aug 07	Johnny Cash 14 Albums 2000 - 2005. 78 Albums part 5 Varios		1.25 GB	22	30
11 Oct 07	Johnny Cash American Recordings I-V [Stumac75]FLAC]		1.21 GB	24	50
27 Aug 07	Johnny Cash - 12 Albums. 1992 - 1999, Various. (5 parts 78 albums) [		1.08 GB	12	52
23 Aug 07	Johnny Cash 15 Albums 1974 1991 -Demonoid com- 1192170 7602		979.15 MB	26	44
07 Aug 07	Johnny Cash - 16 albums, 1968 - 1973		891.19 MB	21	50
29 Jan 07	Country-Johnny Cash-13 cd	1	826.55 MB	1	1
29 Jan 07	Country-Johnny Cash-13 cd		824.51 MB	3	4
26 Jul 07	Johnny Cash - 21 Albums, 1956 - 1966		809.5 MB	21	44
14 Nov 06	Johnny Cash - The Last Great American mpg		789.96 MB	1	1
08 Aug 06	Johnny Cash - The Last Great American mpg	1	789.96 MB	64	5
08 Jan 07	Johnny Cash The Unauthorised Biography 2006 DVDRip XviD-aAF	2	705.74 MB	1	1
07 Dec 06	Johnny Cash Anthology - 15 Clasic Tracks - TV recording		687.94 MB	11	10
23 Jan 07	Johnny Cash - Man In Black (The Very Best Of) (2002) [FLAC][Colombo-bt.org]	1	687.39 MB	157	36
29 Jan 07	Country-Johnny Cash-11 cd		628.11 MB	1	3
09 Feb 07	Johnny Cash - 11 Albums		626.42 MB	0	108
29 Jan 07	Johnny Cash - 11 cd		626.42 MB	2	2
15 Mar 06	Johnny Cash in San Quentin (1969)		584.41 MB	0	2
01 Mar 06	Johnny Cash in San Quentin (1969)		584.32 MB	1	1
12 Sep 07	Johnny Cash - Unearthed 5 CD's (MP3@320kbps)		556.45 MB	1	2
17 Jul 07	Johnny Cash - Unearthed 5 CD's (MP3@320kbps)		556.44 MB	20	12
01 Sep 07	Johnny Cash - Unearthed 5 CD's (MP3@320Kbps)[www funfile org]		556.44 MB	3	1
17 May 06	Johnny Cash 1960-64		545.66 MB	1	4
11 Dec 06	Johnny Cash - Live at Montreux - 1994 - TV recording		531.43 MB	3	1
10 Dec 06	Johnny Cash - Live at Montreux - 1994 - TV recording		531.41 MB	14	7

Figure 12.1 Results of a BitTorrent search for music from the artist Johnny Cash

It would seem therefore that RAT provides a reasonably sound explanation for the phenomenon of illegal file-sharing. However, when applied more generally to digital crime (and particularly cybercrime) RAT may begin to show its limitations. As Yar (2005a) argues, these limitations become most acute where crimes are enacted in virtual environments. For example, much of RAT is based on the reasonable assumption that the motivated offender and suitable victim must be present at the same time at the same place for a crime to occur. However, for a range of cybercrimes this seems not to be the case as many can be committed at distance and can even (in the example of Trojan viruses) be displaced in time. However, perhaps RAT can after all, be reconciled with the digital era through extending the definitions of targets, offenders and guardians.

Certainly, the notion of a target needs further exploration in terms of cyber-crime. In general, the target in RAT represents in essence an opportunity to commit a crime, and often includes the notion of a victim. For cybercrimes, the oppor-tunity presents itself to a potential offender, but as we have already noted, the harm caused by the offender's actions are very unlikely to take place within the offender's vicinity, and the offender does not have to be in any contact with the victim or the victim's physical possessions. A cybercrime may be effectively extended through time and space. This is of no consequence to the applicability of RAT, once the notion of a target has been narrowed to that of an opportunity, excluding any notion of a victim within the vicinity of the offender. For a potential offender, the victim of a crime merely represents an opportunity to commit a crime. The originators of RAT, Felson and Clarke (1998), explore these ideas more fully.

12.1.2 Social learning theory (differential association)

A pervasive criminological theory, particularly in the US, is Edwin Sutherland's differential association theory, and subsequent revisions of the theory, for example Akers, (1985) under the general heading of 'social learning theory'. According to this paradigm, crime is essentially a learned behaviour and in many senses no different from other more commonplace and socially acceptable examples of learning. Individuals, particularly young people, learn through communicating in groups, and in the early years learning takes place from the immediate group surrounding the child, normally the family. From adolescence onwards, other social groups become more influential, including peer groups. (However, it is important to note that social learning theory is not the same as 'peer group pressure' but is instead a more subtle form of social learning). If a person associates mainly with groups that consider crime as normal and acceptable behaviour, and less frequently with those that consider criminal acts as unacceptable, the person is more likely to adopt the stance of the former than the latter. Hence 'differential association' underpins the rationale for the theory. In terms of crime, this learning from others refers to not only more general forms of learning, but also to the acquisition of knowledge about how to commit certain kinds of criminal activity.

Superficially, differential association would seem to be a promising explanation for some forms of digital crime. Yar (2005b) for example, has described how youth involvement in hacking may be conceptualised within differential association, and empirical research (Higgins, 2006) demonstrated that social learning theory (out of the five theories tested) provided the best explanation for 'digital piracy' amongst a non-random sample of undergraduates in the US. The availability of materials containing extreme violence and pornography on the internet has been associated with a normalisation of such activities and has been blamed for a claimed increase in violent and sexual crimes. Certainly, the illegal downloading of copyrighted music from the internet has become so widespread that it is perceived as a normal rather than as an illegal activity.

Parts of the internet are very much made up of 'groups', such as usenet, Google groups, blogs, forums and FaceBook, providing new opportunities for differential association with no geographical limitations. In August 2007 there were over 10 000 Google groups in the English language alone (Google, 2007). Many of the groups are based on special interests, most of which are entirely legal in outlook; however some social groups operating on the internet are undoubtedly used to communicate and share information relating to digital crimes, such as how to commit satellite piracy. As we noted in Chapter 7, the security of the encryption techniques used by a number of European satellite TV providers has been compromised allowing illegal and free access to their services. An added dimension for UK viewers is that many of the European providers broadcast hardcore adult pornography, not available through domestic satellite services. There are three main approaches used to gain unofficial access and circumvent the access control mechanisms; changing the firmware of the receiver itself (if possible), using a modified CAM (conditional access module) or using unofficial smartcards, and combinations of all three approaches are also possible. Internet forum groups are used openly to discuss the techniques involved; how to access codes for downloading and the counter-measures used by the companies to protect their services. The hosts of these forums however, are normally careful to emphasise (usually in capital letters) that 'NO KEYS, BINS OR HEX FILES TO BE POSTED' presumably in order to avoid action by the satellite companies concerned. For the same reason the names of various encryption standards such as Seca or Viacess are replaced within the forums with S*ca or other forms of modified spelling in order to avoid automated detection. Hence this social learning about satellite TV piracy is reinforced by the need to also adopt (or at least to understand) specialised subcultural languages.

Social learning theory would therefore seem to provide a persuasive explanation for at least some forms of behaviour leading to digital crime, and particularly satellite TV (and perhaps more general forms) hacking. However, social learning theory limitations when applied to digital crime mirror its more general limitations. For example, differential association in particular offers no explanation for why in superficially similar circumstances some people choose to 'learn' deviant behaviour whilst others do not (Newburn, 2007, p.152). Part of the explanation might be that a person is not merely a passive recipient of his or her environment; it is not hard to see that many people play an active role in creating their environment. After all, given the nature of the internet, with its huge volume of information and resources, most would-be satellite TV hackers would presumably need to actively seek out hacking-related information and those with similar interests. It is unlikely that, considering the specialist nature of the activity, that 'proto' satellite TV hackers will differentially associate with existing and active hackers by chance alone.

12.1.3 Labelling

As Tierney (2006, p.140) notes, labelling is less of a theory and more of a perspective on crime. That is, it tends to offer explanations for why certain sequences of events occur, rather than providing an underpinning theoretical structure. Labelling perspectives owe much to the work of Howard Becker in the 1960s and 1970s, and although rarely discussed now in their original form, their ideas still find expression in more recent criminological theory.

Hacker Labels

Robin Bryant

Hacking may provide a good example of labelling theory in action. In the early days of computing the term 'hacker' had few of its current negative connotations. Indeed, it appears that it may have been used in a positive way, implying some degree of respect for the skilful hacker who was able to coax an unsuccessful program into some kind of life or devise an innovative solution to a particular problem. Over time there has been a gradual shift in the meaning of the term 'hacker', and it now embraces some of the now more familiar anti-social and illegal dimensions of hacking. There has also been a proliferation in descriptive terms within hacking itself; some of these are summarised in figure 12.2 below.

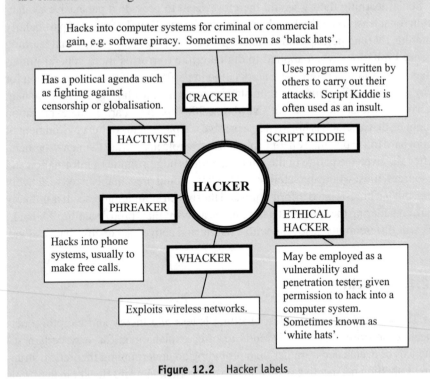

Figure 12.2   Hacker labels

A fundamental premise of labelling is that it is the response to a particular behaviour (rather than the behaviour itself) that leads to a behaviour being labelled as 'deviant'. In everyday terms, 'deviance is in the eye of the beholder'. In addition, if the actions of an individual are identified as being deviant (although perhaps, no different from many other people's) the individual themselves may be labelled as a 'deviant'. In this way, those identified as performing criminal acts become known as 'criminals', and furthermore, their experience of the criminal justice system and the attendant punishment and 'shaming' only serve to reinforce the labelling. This has the further effect of alienating the people concerned and extenuating and perpetuating the deviant behaviour (Merton's 'self fulfilling prophecy').

Until relatively recently, telephone systems in many countries used a simple 'tone' dial system to route calls (rather than the more sophisticated DTMF now used). The frequency of the sound would represent a number or other forms of information. So for example, in the US a tone with frequency 2600 Hz was used to 'reset' a long distance call, permitting further calls to be made through the same line. As noted in previous chapters, devices were built (often referred to as 'Blue Boxes') which would emulate the tones used. After phoning a free long-distance number in the normal way, the device could be used to reset the line (a procedure not normally available to members of the public), and the line could then be used to make further long-distance calls, free of charge.

An early developer and user of Blue Boxes in the US was Steve Wozniak, co-founder of Apple Computers, who also learned how to make them and also sold them to fellow students (Wozniak and Smith, 2006). Later Wozniak recollected that:

> The early boxes had a safety feature – a reed switch inside the housing operated by a magnet taped onto the outside of the box. If apprehended, you removed the magnet, whereupon it would generate off-frequency tones and be inoperable [...] and you tell the police: It's just a music box (cited by Computer History Museum, 2007).

Wozniak's actions are now viewed as examples of his portentous grasp of new technology, his understanding of the landscape of the digital world and his innovative and entrepreneurial style. He was not presumably 'labelled' at the time, or subsequently, in a way that may have led him in a different career direction.

The activity of unauthorised accessing of telecommunication systems (illegal in many countries) has become known as 'phreaking'. (The *Oxford English Dictionary* traces the use of the term to a 1971 article in a US magazine. Presumably it was a conflation of the words 'phoning' and 'freak' as the word freak was used at the time as a term to describe eccentric intellectual types.) The relatively benign view now apparently taken of Wozniak's early hacking activities stands in marked contrast to the judgement meted out to his modern day equivalents in the UK; in 1999, a 20-year-old man received a 2-year suspended sentence at Southwark Crown Court in London for 'phreaking' a Nicaraguan telephone exchange and making free international calls (BBC, 1999). The judge described him as an 'absolute menace' (BBC, 1999).

12.2 Motivational perspectives

In this section we examine motivational aspects of digital crime, illustrated through a consideration of the phenomenon of 'hacking'.

Stereotypically, the notion of the hacker tends to call to mind images of teenage boys sitting alone in their bedrooms, tapping away at a keyboard in attempt to become one of the L33T H4X0R5 (elite hackers). Historically, this image had some credence in the early days of public network access (Sterling, 1992) when specialist skills and equipment were required to join the electronic community. With the advent of the internet as a public resource, however, the ubiquity of commoditised equipment and software (such as ADSL and user-friendly web browsers) has created the opportunity for anyone to join the community, and has radically transformed the nature of the online community from an exclusive club populated by knowledgeable users into a reflection of the wider global community.

In the early days, most cybercrime seems to have been confined to classical 'hacking' or exploration of the limits of software, hardware and the hacker him/herself. Hackers tended to be motivated by a desire to prove or test oneself against the 'high priests' of the networked world and very little of it was malicious. Successful hackers, therefore, were rewarded with high self-esteem and peer-group recognition as members of a very exclusive club.

As the number of users on the network increased however, the number of potential victims increased, along with the number of crimes which could be adapted for use within the new environment.

As noted in Chapter 1, from the criminals' perspective the internet provides a fair degree of anonymity, coupled with the ability to reach a large number of victims very quickly at low cost. These two factors also prove attractive to those who would not consider carrying out a criminal act in person, because of the risk of being caught during a face to face transaction.

As an example, we could consider Rogers' (2000) taxonomy of hackers, the key features of which are summarised in Table 12.2.

Table 12.2 A taxonomy of hackers

Hacker category	Motivation	Skills
Newbie/toolkit		Limited skills, limited experience, reliant on others' tools
Cyber-punks	Deliberately attack/ vandalise	Some skills, can create own tools
Internals	Disgruntled or malicious	Insiders with privileged access
Coders		High skill levels
Old guard hackers	No criminal intent, disrespect for personal property	High skill levels
Professional criminals	Motivated by 'profit'	High skill levels, well-equipped
Cyber-terrorists	Motivated by 'ideals'	High skill levels, well-equipped

From Rogers (2000).

'Rogers (2000) goes on to review the research into the motivations of the 'cyber-punk' category of hacker. It would appear from the research that media stereotypes of cyber-punks have some basis in reality; the protagonists are usually young, male and socially isolated, and their actions appear to be motivated by revenge against society and the need to gain a sense of power. The motivations of other categories of hacker appear more concrete, such as financial gain.

12.3 Cyberprofiling

As we argued in section 12.2 above, because of the different motivations for engaging in online crime, and the huge population now involved in internet activity, it is now difficult to describe a 'typical' cybercriminal (such as a hacker) in simple and singular terms. 'Cyberprofiling' attempts to adapt psychological and geographic profiling methods to tackle the problems of identifying and classifying online activity, and to elucidate its likely pattern of propagation together with its perpetrators (Marshall *et al.*, 2005).

Starting with a consideration of RAT (see section 12.1 above), a model of cybercrime has been produced which identifies the key elements required for a cybercrime to succeed.

In this model, six major elements required for a cybercrime are identified:

- A criminal.

- A criminal's 'home' network (the immediate digital and physical environment).

- A victim.

- A victim's 'home' network (the immediate digital and physical environment).

- The internet (or other network used as a means of attack).

- An attack.

Further, it is hypothesised that the relative likelihood that an attack will succeed (L, the attack success quotient) will be a function of the variables C_e, C_f, A, V_e, V_g and C_g (Table 12.3).

That is, the hypothesis is that:

$$L = f(C_e, C_f, A, V_e, V_g, C_g)$$

where f represents a mathematical function of the variables concerned.

Table 12.3   Cyberprofiling variables

Variable	Descriptor
C_e	The criminal's *experience* and *expertise*
C_f	The criminal's *freedom* to move through the public network to cause the attack
A	The nature of the *attack* in terms of prevalence, novelty, robustness, etc.
V_e	The victim's *experience* and *expertise*
V_g	The *guardianship* of a *victim* (measures designed to protect the victim within the 'home' network)
C_g	The *guardianship* of the *criminal* (measures designed to stop the criminal acting beyond his or her 'home' network)

As an example, we could consider Rogers' (2000) taxonomy of hackers, described in section 12.2 above.

The 'newbies' clearly have low ratings for C_e whereas the professional criminals and terrorists will have very high C_e values. Similarly, attacks launched by newbies are likely to have a low rating for A as they are dependent on existing tools and methods, whereas the professional and terrorist groups are highly motivated and skilled enough to generate entirely new types of attack with a high A rating.

Some of the properties of the criminal (e.g. the motive for committing the crime) may be the result of attacks on those criminals, leading to the possibility of a chain of precursor offences which can be discovered and examined through the use of this approach.

One working model of the function f is to model L as being directly related to the product of C_e, C_f and A but inversely related to the product of V_e, V_g and a power of C_g; that is of the form:

$$L = (C_e \times C_f \times A)/(V_e \times V_g \times C_g^x)$$

where x is an index (to be determined) of C_g, representing the experience that well-designed networks do not allow attacks to escape. This would suggest that the guardianship of the criminal's home network may have more mathematical significance than any other factor.

Within this working model, the variables C_e, C_f, A, V_e, V_g and C_g are allocated integer values between 1 and 5 inclusive, where 1 represents a low estimate and 5 a high; the exact value of x (which may be non-integer) in a number of examples is currently being determined through statistical techniques such as multinomial logistic regression (Marshall *et al.*, 2005).

The higher the resulting value of L, the greater the chance that a cyberattack will succeed. Application of this formula, using appropriate estimates, allows the likelihood of success of a particular attack to be calculated in comparison with other attacks. Where elements have unknown values, the function can be analysed to provide estimates of the unknown values and thus help to generate profiles of the missing elements.

The model may also be applied to specific examples of digital crime, particularly cybercrime. Within the following examples, the working model described above has been used, and the value of x here is 2.

Example 1 – Portable digital music device fraud

In this fraud a portable digital device (such as an iPod) is apparently offered for sale on an online auction site (such as eBay) for a very small cost, such as 99p. The reality is that the successful bidder has actually bought only the information (often in the form of an ebook or URL) about 'How to buy an iPod' rather than the device itself. Typically the offenders will use long and complex descriptions of the goods in order to mask the underlying deception. An analysis of the language used by offenders strongly suggests that they are young and/or inexperienced (Marshall *et al.*, 2005).

In this case we may reasonably allocate numerical values to the variables as follows:

C_e = moderate, estimated as 3.

C_f = high, 5 (using the internet, which is inherently insecure).

A = moderate, estimated as 3 (well constructed, not rare but new to the victim).

V_e = low, estimated as 1 (only younger or naïve and inexperienced auction house users are likely to be conned).

V_g = low, 1 (significant supervision of the victim's home network is unlikely).

C_g = low, estimated as 1 (typically a home network, such as bedroom PC linked to a modem and router).

Hence in this example, the attack success quotient is $L = (3 \times 5 \times 3)/(1 \times 1 \times 1^2) = 45$.

Example 2 – Distributed denial of service attack

A denial of service (DoS) attack is an internet-mediated attempt to 'bring down' a website or other internet service or resource (such as a DNS server), normally through quickly and repeatedly sending 'packets' of data which are intended to overwhelm the target. Distributed Denial of service (DDoS) attacks are coordinated DoS attacks from multiple locations, perhaps using 'zombies' or 'bots' secretly inhabiting and using the PCs of other unsuspecting internet users. For example, by sending millions of almost simultaneous requests for the same webpage an organisation's servers may be overwhelmed and subsequently crash. DDoS attacks are conducted for a number of reasons (including political motives) but are also used to conduct criminal acts (such as extortion or revenge). As discussed earlier in Chapter 2, DDoS attacks are now illegal in the UK, following amendments to the Computer Misuse Act 1990 by the Police and Justice Act 2006.

Conducting a DDoS requires some technical knowledge, organisational skills and significant levels of preparation on part of the perpetrators. Therefore, in terms of the model described above, the following may be used as suitable values for the variables in the case of DDoS attacks:

C_e = high, 5 (established and experienced offenders).

C_f = high, 4 (as in the previous example, for this crime the internet is inherently insecure).

A = low or moderate, say 2 (although DDoS attacks are relatively common and the dangers widely discussed, they may also be new to a particular victim and be inherently difficult to avoid or prevent).

V_e = low, 2 (there is currently a significant lack of expertise and experience amongst potential victims).

V_g = moderate, 3 (there are numerous hardware and software firewalls and anti-virus programs to help guard against DDoS).

C_g = low, 1 (unlikely to have any controls in place).

Hence in this example, the attack success prediction quotient is $L = (5 \times 4 \times 2)/(2 \times 3 \times 1^2) = 6.66$ (recurring).

Example 3 – Physical CD piracy

As discussed in Chapter 1, physical CD piracy involves the large-scale illegal copying of commercially produced CDs for distribution and sale to third parties. Copying facilities might be based in a person's home or (in the case of more organised criminals) even in a factory. Physical CD piracy requires both equipment and supplies but both are relatively easy to source, and the technical expertise involved is of a low level. However, distribution of the pirated CDs and the recovery of profits may prove particularly challenging for the criminals involved; these activities tend to be the hallmarks of more organised and specialist criminals.

This suggests the following possible values for the variables:

C_e = low, a value of 1 (hardware and software easily sourced and operated).

C_f = medium, 3 (could be halted at any time, particularly during the sales process).

$A =$ low, 2 (CD piracy is well known and is not new).

$V_e =$ high, 4 (significant industry knowledge, and experience of countering CD piracy).

$V_g =$ high, 4 (the industry is motivated through self-interest, with its own investigatory capability).

$C_g =$ medium, 3 (CD piracy needs space, equipment used is easy to identify).

Hence in this case $L = (1 \times 3 \times 2)/(4 \times 4 \times 3^2) = 0.042$.

12.3.1 Discussion of examples

In summary, the likelihood of a successful attack for each of our examples is:

- Portable digital music device fraud, 45; and hence very likely.
- DDoS attack, 6.67; and hence likely.
- Physical CD piracy, 0.042; that is easy to perpetrate but unlikely to succeed.

The importance of these results does not lie in their absolute numerical values (calculated as they are, from one particular working model) but in the relative order derived and their potential use as a predictive device. In the same way that the 'CRAVED' model discussed in Chapter 1 may be employed to assess the 'stealability' of new consumer goods in advance of their commercial introduction, so cyberprofiling has the potential to be used to help determine the likely impact of new digital crimes.

Although the model can be applied manually, working on a case by case basis, the sheer volume of online activity means that it is perhaps desirable for it to be automated to enable severe attacks to be detected early and 'nuisance' activity to be blocked or ignored as appropriate.

Questions

Robin Bryant & Sarah Bryant

1. What arguments have been put forward in support of the idea that some crime 'problems' are being socially constructed in the era of the internet?

2. Are there examples of Stanley Cohen's 'Moral Panics' to be found in reactions to digital crime?

3. To what extent can the unauthorised use of a domestic wireless network be accounted for by routine activity theory?

4. List, with reasons, three digital crimes that might be partly explained by 'differential association'.

5. How could we explain using labelling theory the reasons why a 'script-kiddie' might move on to commit more serious types of digital crime?

6. A hacking attack might or might not succeed. When attempting to assess the chances of the attack succeeding, what factors may need to be taken into account associated with (a) a potential hacker, and (b) the potential victim?

7. A mathematical equation is proposed in section 12.3. How could the accuracy of its predictive power be assessed?

References

Akers, R. (1985) *Deviant Behaviour: A Social Learning Approach*. Belmont: Wadsworth.

BBC (1999) Phone hacker dials £106 000 bill. BBC News [Online]. Available at: http://news.bbc.co.uk/1/hi/uk/469248.stm (Accessed: Oct 11 2007).

BBC (2005) Legal fight hits 'music pirates'. BBC News [Online]. Available at: http://news.bbc.co.uk/1/hi/entertainment/music/4438324.stm (Accessed: Oct 11 2007).

Burke, R. (2005) *An Introduction to Criminological Theory*. Cullompton: Willan Publishing.

Clarke, R.V. and Felson, M. (1993) Routine activity and rational choice. In: Clarke, R.V. & Felson, M. (eds.) *Advances in Criminological Theory* Vol. 5: *Routine Activity and Rational Choice*. New Brunswick, NJ: Transaction Press, pp. 17–36.

Computer History Museum (2007) Timeline of Computer History 1972. [Online]. Available at: http://www.computerhistory.org/timeline/?year=1972 (Accessed: Oct 11 2007).

Farrell, G. and Pease, K. (2006) Criminology and security. In: Gill, M. (ed.) *Handbook of Security*. Basingstoke: Macmillan.

Felson, M. and Clarke, R. (eds.) (1998) Opportunity makes the thief: practical theory for crime prevention. In: Webb, B. (ed.) *Police Research Series* Paper 98.

Google (2007) Group directory All groups Language: English. [Online]. Available at: http://groups.google.co.uk/groups/dir?lnk=odl&hl=en&sel=67188898 (Accessed: 11 Oct 2007).

Higgins, G. (2006) Digital piracy: assessing the contributions of an integrated self-control theory and social learning theory using structural equation modelling. *Criminal Justice Studies*, **19**(1):3–22.

Home Office (2006) Routine activity theory. [Online]. Available at: http://www.crimereduction.gov.uk/skills/skills08.htm (Accessed: Oct 11 2007).

Jaishankar, K. (2007) Cyber criminology: Evolving a novel discipline with a new journal *International Journal of Cyber Criminology* **1**(1):1–6.

Maguire, M., Morgan, R. and Reiner, R. (eds.) (2007) *Oxford Handbook of Criminology*, 4th edition. Oxford: Oxford University Press.

Marshall, A.M., Tompsett, B.C. and Semmens, N.C. (2005) Cyberprofiling: offender and geographic profiling of crime on the Internet. Proceedings of the Workshop of the 1st International Conference on Security and Privacy for Emerging Areas in Communication Networks, IEEE, 2005, pp. 21–24.

Newburn, T. (2007) *Criminology.* Cullompton: Willan Publishing.

Rogers, M. (2000) A New Hacker Taxonomy. University of Manitoba, [Online] Available at: http://homes.cerias.purdue.edu/~mkr/hacker.doc (Accessed: Oct 10 2007).

Sterling, B. (1992) The Hacker Crackdown: Law and Disorder on the Electronic Frontier New York: Viking.

Tierney, J. (2006) *Criminology: Theory and Context*, 2nd edition. Harlow: Pearson Education Ltd.

Wall, D. (2007) *Cybercrime.* Cambridge: Polity Press.

Wozniak, S. and Smith, G. (2006) *iWoz: Computer Geek to Cult Icon: Getting to the Core of Apple's Inventor*. London: Headline Review.

Yar, M. (2005a) The novelty of 'cybercrime' an assessment in light of routine activity theory. *European Journal of Criminology* **2**(4):407–427.

Yar, M. (2005b) Computer hacking: just another case of juvenile delinquency? *The Howard Journal* **44**(4):387–399.

Index

Note: Page references in *italics* refer to Figures: those in **bold** refer to Tables

Investigating Digital Crime   Edited by Robin Bryant and Sarah Bryant
© 2008 John Wiley & Sons, Ltd

Index compiled by Annette Musker